The Best Health Ideas I Know

The Best Health Ideas I Know

including My Personal Plan
for Living

by Robert Rodale

Published by Rodale Press Book Division
Emmaus, Pennsylvania 18049

Book design by Donald E. Breter
Jacket photographs by Tom Gettings

International Standard Book Number 0-87857-082-9
Library of Congress Card Number 73-21133

PRINTED IN THE UNITED STATES OF AMERICA
Printed on recycled paper

FIRST PRINTING—June, 1974

SECOND PRINTING—September, 1974

THIRD PRINTING—November, 1974

FOURTH PRINTING—January, 1975

PB 421

CONTENTS

HEALTH IS A TALENT 1

The first step to improved health is to learn what health really is. Many of us have picked up a grab-bag assortment of impressions concerning the subject from advertising, promotion campaigns and other propaganda. The result is that totally erroneous ideas about health abound, and many people are unwitting "health cripples." These unfortunates go through life in a kind of one-dimensional way— missing out on the exciting and pleasurable benefits that true health understanding can give.

A key to this confusion is the way the word "health" is misused.

Almost all of us buy "health" insurance. In reality we are buying insurance against illness. As long as we are healthy, the policy is of no value whatever, except in case of pregnancy. Only when health fails does the real value of the insurance become apparent.

Hospitals are frequently called health centers. Actually, their main function is to cope with disease, illness, and body malfunctions. It is true that many people go into hospitals sick and come out in a better state of health, but it is a long jump from that to saying that hospitals represent the total answer to health challenges. They most certainly don't.

Another example of word misuse is the so-called "health" examination. What it reveals is whether you are sick, not whether you are truly healthy. Our medical system, even including the most exhaustive and "complete" examinations, primarily emphasizes the idea that health is an absence of disease. There is far more to health than simply not being sick.

In addition to these specific ways in which the word health is linked misleadingly to medical concepts, there are many indirect but no less effective assaults on our awareness of what true health means. Medicine advertising is perhaps the best example. There is now a different pill available for almost every physical or mental problem which can afflict man. Although the word health is not always used in promoting these medicines, there is always the strong implication that the use of such pills and potions leads to health. But that's not true!

Almost all medicines in common use—whether sold over the counter or by prescription—merely relieve symptoms. And many times, in the course of relieving symptoms, they cause side effects which are equally troublesome or they lead to addiction problems, creating bad habits which last for a lifetime. In a vast majority of cases, the natural recuperative powers of the body itself conquer disease, in spite of, not because of, the medicines that have been taken. Yet the person who uses medicines is left with the idea that somehow the medicines will promote health by curing, when what they will probably do (if one is fortunate) is to make life a little more bearable while the natural healing process occurs.

Despite all this distortion of the meaning of health, both the word and the concept retain an amazing value and sales appeal. "If you've got your health, you've got just about everything," the attractive, middle-aged actress intones in a TV commercial. Even the rather negative idea that being healthy means not being sick has a powerful attraction to the average person. How much more potent the word health would be if all the abuses were cleared away, and health was presented only as the gloriously positive concept that it is!

The best way to understand the meaning of health is to realize that it is a talent, just as singing, dancing, talking, or sewing is the expression of talent. Let's think about singing, just to cite one example. Everyone who has a voice can sing in some fashion, even if he only croaks out a few off tune notes. But some people work to develop that talent through study and practice. They often get both enjoyment and financial reward by learning how to sing better. The life of a good singer is improved in many ways by the successful attempts to perfect that rewarding talent.

The same values apply to health. Some people are born without much health talent. They are sickly, and often have to go through life struggling against debility. Others are born with a body and mind of incredible strength and efficiency, and can break all the common-sense rules and still live to extreme old age in good health.

No matter what health resources you were born with, you can improve what you have. Actually, improving your health is remarkably easy, once you make up your mind that you want to do it. In fact, the basic rules of health promotion have been known for thousands of years. Do everything in moderation. Avoid rich foods. Get plenty of rest. Get some exercise during each day. "Work up a sweat once a day," a rule the Spartan soldiers followed.

Unfortunately, the simplicity and common sense of the health building idea doesn't automatically sell to more than 10 percent-or-so of the population.

These people are commonly called health nuts, faddists and other unflattering names. I think of this 10 percent as health enthusiasts—excited about developing one of the most important and rewarding of all talents, health. Health enthusiasts are great people, far wiser and happier than the run-of-the-mill citizens who can't seem to mobilize themselves to do anything long-range about their health. Even the act of taking food supplements—the easiest of all health-building techniques—is too much trouble for some.

I am convinced that the way to get the job of health-building done is by helping the public to understand what health really is. Once the true nature of health is understood, people will start to educate themselves about nutrition, fitness, environmental improvement—the building blocks of better health. On that foundation, the structure of motivation can be built. The effort to improve becomes routine, and each success adds to the pleasure of life. Even working hard to become healthier is fun. And finding easy ways to build health talents is sheer joy.

What Is Health?

We agree, I assume, that health is not merely the absence of disease. But let's not try to define a concept as important as health in a few words. The idea is simply too big for that. I can think of at least eight separate components of true health—and each one in some way represents a talent that can be developed. Here is my list:

1. Better health means *greater personal efficiency*. How do you feel? Are you satisfied with the amount of pep and energy you have? Do you adapt to stress easily? Can you get plenty of work done during the day, and still have the desire and energy left to do more in the evening, or do you simply col-

lapse in front of the television set after dinner?

These are questions that bear heavily on your state of health. They are almost never asked during medical examinations, because they may be considered too mundane, too simple to concern medical specialists. Yet such a thing as simply feeling good most of the time is what life—and health—is all about.

What good is it to live without symptoms of disease, if you struggle through your days and evenings in a kind of personal smog? Haven't you ever wondered what it would be like to feel better than you normally do—to be more alert, more observant, to be able to relax easily, and to be able to keep going after others tire?

2. A *better mental situation* is part of the real health I'm talking about. No field of human studies is as complex and controversial as mental health, yet that should not stop you from looking upon your own mind as a fertile field for self-improvement. Nutrition definitely has an effect on the mind, as recent vitamin studies show. Eventually, some of the most troublesome mental illnesses may yield to meganutrition techniques—giving people very large amounts of certain nutrients.

Other, simpler measures can have a strong effect on mental efficiency. For example, a diet low in sugar helps to protect against the low-blood-sugar problem (hypoglycemia) in susceptible people. A switch to natural food, free of additives, has been found to minimize behavior problems in hyperkinetic children. It has been shown that many of the pesticides, additives, and environmental pollutants have an effect on the behavior of experimental animals. Isn't it logical to assume that these factors can be having a similar effect on us, especially after many years of exposure?

Many people cope with mental problems simply by resorting to alcohol or drugs. What they are after is a different way of feeling and thinking. The health enthusiast is seeking the same thing, but he uses natural, more effective and far safer methods to achieve his goal. Alcohol and tranquilizers deaden normal mental functions, but people who turn themselves on to a more healthful way of life say that their minds become clearer, that they feel more alive mentally than ever before. "Life couldn't be better," is a frequently-heard comment. You don't hear that kind of talk from the steady drinkers or pilltakers.

3. Real health means a *slower aging process.* Here is a fantastically interesting area for health improvement. There is no doubt that individuals suffer the effects of increasing age at different rates—even though their chronological age may be the same. We can see it among our friends. Some are weakened by hardened arteries and emphysema by the time they are 50 or even earlier, while others keep bounding along with youthful vigor well into their 70's.

The difference in the rate at which individuals age stems primarily from the way they live—lifestyles and lifetime health are closely related. The person who builds a reasonable amount of diet moderation, physical activity and other sensible health habits into his or her life reaps large benefits in youthfulness later. Those who get their health information from patent-medicine ads generally find themselves slowing down or even conking out well before their time.

Researchers are now beginning to measure the rate at which people age by keeping track of a long list of factors which limit human efficiency. By watching such things as the rates at which weight and blood pressure increase, how and when lung efficiency declines, and even the rate at which hair turns grey, scientists can quickly relate different health techniques to their effect on human efficiency at various ages. As this work proceeds and bears fruit, we are going to see more emphasis on a person's true age—as represented by how he or she can actually enjoy life—and less concern about a mere date on a birth certificate.

4. *Physical fitness* is a good measure of true health. It is also the easiest, most effective way to increase your health talent. Today the average person lives such a sedentary life, and the body's physical mechanisms have been allowed to decline to such an extent that even the simplest, most moderate exercise program can have dramatic beneficial results. For example, I am convinced that nine out of ten people could actually reduce their true age (as measured by an efficiency index) by five to ten years just by walking half an hour a day, every day.

Fitness is so important to health, in fact, that it is almost impossible to draw a real distinction between health in its positive, talent-oriented sense and its physical sense. No person is a more representative "picture of health" than the firm-bodied, middle-aged enthusiast for cycling, running, swimming or hiking. His capacity to do things is so much greater than that of the ordinary person that I know no better way to suggest that you seek true health than by at least trying to follow his example.

You don't have to become dedicated to sports or even to fitness to achieve that benefit. All you have to do is to become physically active again in a gentle but regular way, moving those joints, stretching those muscles, and starting those "juices" flowing. Search again for that wonderful glow that comes when your body has been warmed up by movement. Relish the feeling of ease of action that results. That's health!

5. *Resistance to infection,* and quicker recov-

ery, are marks of genuine health. How well you can resist cold germs, and other viruses and "bugs," is not the kind of thing that is revealed by a medical examination, yet it is an excellent index of your health status. To appreciate that fully, though, you have to realize that germs don't really "cause" disease. If they really did, everyone would be sick all the time, because disease-causing microorganisms are present almost everywhere. They are simply the agents of disease, and multiply only in people who are peculiarly susceptible at any given moment.

True, resistance created by antibodies and inoculations can be important protection against contagious disease, but other factors come into play which aren't yet completely understood. Why do people who take large amounts of vitamin C suffer less from the effects of colds? We don't know. Why do women who wear intrauterine birth control devices made of copper have a certain degree of immunity against venereal disease? We don't know. Why are some people "always getting sick" while others who live in a similar environment rarely miss work? We don't know.

While the specific factors that create this immunity remain to be pinpointed, it is known that a person's general level of health plays an extremely important role. This immunity to contagious sickness can be increased by developing your health talent through improved diet, enhanced fitness, and other means.

Natural, health-oriented resistance to disease will soon be much more important than it is now, if for no other reason than the fact that the antibiotics and other "miracle drugs" on which people have come to rely are rapidly losing their impact. They have been sadly overused, causing a great many people to develop dangerous sensitivities and allowing many kinds of bacteria to become immune to their effects. Strains of disease organisms that cannot be curbed by antibiotics now inhabit and thrive in most hospitals. Roughly 20 percent of those who enter hospitals for any reason contract infections from these drug resistant organisms. According to one recent estimate close to 100,000 people die from such infections each year. You can readily see, therefore, how important it is to develop a strong talent for staying away from infection—and out of hospitals.

6. Health talent and *beauty* go together. Sure, people who aren't handsome or beautiful can possess remarkable health. But though they aren't fashion models, there is a glow of vitality radiating from them that all who aspire to good looks wish they had. And it goes without saying that anyone who wants exceptional beauty must use every conceivable health-building idea to lay a solid foundation for good appearance. The widespread health-consciousness among actors and actresses is evidence of that. And they get results!

A good figure is the starting point of any beauty program, and healthful diet coupled with regular exercise is the way to achieve this goal. There is, actually, no natural way to beautify your body without also making progress toward better health.

Attractive skin, also vital to beauty, is another yardstick of health. Here again, the very techniques which enhance skin beauty increase health too. Proper diet is important, so are cleanliness, avoiding pollution, and guarding against excessive exposure to the sun. Too much sun can lead to early wrinkling and even skin cancer.

Hair beauty is another bonus in building health. Proper mineral nutrition is particularly reflected in the improved quality and appearance of the hair. While there's no way that I know to escape the genetic handicap of male pattern baldness, many can

9

improve the quality of whatever hair they have by becoming healthier. That's just one more good reason to aim for real health.

7. *Sexual vitality* is another index of health talent. While we all recognize that the world is over-populated, and I personally am not interested in giving advice that will help you become a sexual athlete, we can't help being aware that the ability to perform the sex act with real joy and effectiveness is an index of health. And those who can retain that ability into advanced old age deserve our admiration and respect.

The Abkhasians in Russia, some of whom live to be over 125 years old, routinely perform their marital functions to the age of 100. The Hunzas become parents at advanced ages, and so do the residents of Vilcabamba, that mountain valley in Equador known for the extreme old age its residents reach. There is no reason why we can't adapt our lifestyles to gain the health advantages these remarkable people enjoy.

How is it done? There are no tricks, no aphrodisiacs. Even if true aphrodisiacs did exist, how could they stimulate your sexual function past the age of 100, if illness had snuffed out your life at 55? We can only look at the way of life these long-living, sexually active people follow, and see what we can copy.

The Abkhasians have an abhorrence of stale food. Everything is prepared fresh for each meal. Members of all three long-lived societies eat much less than we do, and their food is simple and unprocessed.Yet, despite meager diets, they work harder physically. Their bodies are lean and hard, not larded with fat.

Certain vitamins and trace minerals contained in the traditional foods these people eat could play an important role. Vitamin E is present in liberal amounts in the unprocessed, whole grains common to their diets. They could also be eating food rich in zinc, now known to be closely associated both with growth and normal sexual function. Other still-un-identified mineral factors could also be involved.

Only one thing is absolutely certain. The talent for health and the talent for sexual potency in later life are branches of the same tree.

8. *Continuous challenge* is the final element in a talent for health. There is no limit to how healthy you can become. This same uncertainty about maxi-mum achievement is associated with the develop-ment of any talent. You can always keep moving to-ward perfection, yet you never really get there. Rec-ords are made to be broken, as they say in sports.

Proof of the concept that health is a talent lies in the unlimited challenge that the search for health presents. Once you learn the true nature of health, you have room to expand your consciousness, to reach for personal greatness, or just to wave your arms in happy abandon if that suits your mood. You are fi-nally free of the constricting idea that health is some-thing you get in a drug packet, or as a reward for al-lowing a doctor to operate on you. The power to be healthy, you finally realize, is largely in your own hands.

MY PERSONAL PLAN FOR HEALTHFUL LIVING 2

The public has every right to be curious about the kind of health system I follow in my own life. After all, I continually suggest how others can improve *their* health, so why shouldn't they want to know whether I take that advice myself?

There are other reasons why I want to tell my personal story—about how I control my weight, handle my health problems, motivate myself to exercise, and so forth. For one thing, by learning about what I do, you might better understand some of your own health challenges. You can see which aspects of health I consider most important; and, in my "case history" you can see how all the different facets of a natural plan for health work when applied in the life of one person. That could be very helpful in deciding which health improvement techniques might be most beneficial to you.

I was brought up in a health-conscious family, which is a big help in getting a young person started off on the right foot. My father, J. I. Rodale, was concerned about finding independent ways to help himself to better health even before I was born, in 1930. J. I. hated the thought of being "one of the sheep." He believed that most people blindly follow the crowd more concerned about doing what is popular than in trying to create a way of life suited to their individual needs. He was vitally interested in health improvement; he saw clearly that health is not something you find in the doctor's office or at the drugstore. He continually searched for all kinds of health ideas and didn't hesitate to experiment by changing his diet and doing other things that he thought might cure some of his problems or give him more vitality.

Natural food supplements in tablet or capsule form were not available then, but I can recall gulping many a spoonful of cod liver oil, and not complaining much about the taste, either. Like everyone else we had no money to spare during The Depression, but the lunches I took to school were not the white bread and baloney sandwiches of the other kids. I always got raw vegetables and fruit, and a sandwich of fresh meat on black bread. Never was I given the cupcakes and cookies I saw the others eating, although I do remember buying candy once in a while. Our diet was not an extreme example of health foodism. In fact, until he became aware of the problem of chemical additives, J. I. and the rest of us used to eat a dish of ice cream after supper quite often.

When I was 11, my father bought a worn-out farm a few miles outside of Allentown, Pennsylvania —primarily to have a source of food for our family during the war that everyone expected. In the process of doing that, he discovered and began popularizing the organic system of gardening and farming—which meant that during my teenage years and thereafter I ate a diet of fresh, organically-grown foods.

The farm meant much more than that to me, though. I was soon given chores to do, and was taught much about the craft of farming by the men we got to help us with the work. Mainly, I learned that hard, physical work, the lot of many people on this earth, breeds a sense of self-respect that you can't get any other way. Although I sometimes complained about having to work hard, I now look back on those days with a good deal of pleasure and wish I could live them over again.

As a member of a health minded family I had the feeling that it was normal to be interested in improving your body. I didn't think it was sissy to be health conscious. So when my father told me that I would get sick from smoking cigarettes, I didn't try. But even when quite young I must have had some urge to know more about health—because I can remember earning the personal health and public health merit badges soon after becoming a Boy Scout. My career goal always was to go into writing and publishing, though—not to become a doctor.

Two health problems I had during my youth stick in my mind: Often I was troubled with pains in the feet and legs, which doctors said were caused by bad arches. The pain seemd to hit when I lay down to sleep at night and would be bad enough to keep me awake. My parents massaged my feet and legs, which helped. When I was still quite young, my mother bought me special shoes, which largely controlled the problem. To this day, though, I still find that heavy climbing boots are the only footgear that will prevent foot pain if I have to walk long distances, which I enjoy doing. When I travel I always leave home in a pair of these big shoes, so if you ever see me walking through some airport wearing a pair of five-pound boots, you'll know why. Fortunately, that kind of boot doesn't seem out of place now, and is actually in fashion. To me, they feel even more comfortable than bedroom slippers. The weight helps you move along steadily by turning your legs into pendulums.

15

My other health problem was weight. By the time I was 16 years old I had reached my full height —5 feet 11½ inches—but weighed 199 pounds and had a 35 inch waist. I was "pear shaped," as the fitness experts say today. My upper body was relatively underdeveloped (I worked on the farm only in the summers) and most of my weight was in hips, thighs, and legs. The cause of the problem was simply too much eating and sitting, and not enough regular exercise. The food at home was very good, and I was the clean-up artist.

Today, my weight is 148 pounds—quite a difference! How did I manage to lose over 50 pounds and *stay* slim? Well, it was not done overnight or with any trick diets. Mainly, over the years I became educated about the need to keep weight down and managed to control my appetite as a result. As a young man I can remember eating tremendous amounts of food, and having almost a competitive attitude about how much I could eat. If other people were eating one steak sandwich, I would eat two. The same went for portions of other foods. The word got around that I was a big eater, and I enjoyed that reputation.

Then at the age of 18 I went on a six-week trip to Mexico by myself, and nobody knew or cared how much I ate. I also picked up a case of the tourist disease there, which helped shed a few pounds. At any rate, I came home about 30 pounds lighter, and had to buy all new clothes. Enjoying my new slimness, I consciously tried to eat less and was able to keep my weight down.

Shortly after returning home, I started commuting to a nearby university. I stopped at a diner on the way to have breakfast many mornings. I figured that my weight was so much under control that I could afford to eat some kind of pastry each morning, which I did. I really enjoyed the taste. I had previously reached the conclusion on my own that refined sugar is not a good food, mainly because it does not occur in nature, but has to be processed for regular use in food. I also knew that sugar is fattening.

Within two months, I was ten pounds fatter. Reluctantly, I gave up the morning pastry habit. I didn't want to get in my old fat state again. In another few months I lost the taste for sugared things almost entirely, and didn't even feel I was making a big sacrifice. That experience taught me that if you are aware and motivated, you can wean yourself from the taste of some foods that are detrimental to your health. Probably some people are more affected by what are known as "food cues" than I am, and can't bear to pass a bakery without going inside to buy something. But most people can easily adjust to liking what's good for them.

After marriage, my weight went up again. Young married men are the most rapid weight-gainers, and I was no exception. But again I managed to trim down gradually. Ardie, my wife, says it is because she stopped putting butter on all the vegetables and making rich sauces. Probably she is right, although I do consciously eat small portions of some foods and stay away as much as possible from the butter dish and desserts of all kinds. Today I find weight control no problem at all. In fact I have to tell myself to eat more once in a while, just to bring my weight up a few pounds. That's fortunate because as you get older you need less food to maintain the same weight. I believe almost everyone should trim back on his food intake progressively as he gets older, just to avoid gaining. To actually lose as you age means cutting back on food even more drastically. All the more reason to get your weight to the right level while young.

Although I enjoy eating, I am not like the gourmet who constantly seeks unusual flavors and a tremendous variety of foods. My father always favored simple foods—"one thing at a time on the plate"—as he used to say, and undoubtedly my taste in food was influenced by him. There is nothing wrong with being a gourmet, of course, but I think that if you are going to make food flavor a passion you must also build up your defenses against overweight more strongly than the average person.

My food thrills come not so much from fancy restaurants or dinner-party meals, but from the crisp and natural flavor of salads fresh from an organic garden, or the wonderful taste of fresh-from-the-oven bread made from organic grain.

I eat plenty of fruits, vegetables, nuts (especially peanuts) and foods made from whole grains. They fill you up rather quickly, and keep you filled up for a longer time than the kinds of food that make up the typical American diet.

Most people today focus their diet on meat, refined grains, processed potatoes, snacks, and sugar-loaded foods like pastries, ice cream and candy. While they are good sources of food energy (which is usually not burned up completely) they don't contain enough bulk to provide a feeling of satisfaction for four or five hours. In fact, many processed foods seem to trigger a taste response that calls you to keep on eating and snacking. That is less often the case with natural foods.

Meat is a feature of my diet, but in recent years I have cut down drastically on the size of the portions. I also try to avoid eating meat at breakfast and lunch. My motives are not only ecological (meat requires a lot of energy to produce), but nutritional. Why load yourself up with more calories and fat than you need? Why not get accustomed today to the diet of the future, which is going to be heavy on foods from plants and very light on meat? I do eat five or six eggs a week and moisten my cereal with some skim milk; I eat very little cheese. Most cheeses contain a lot of salt and fat, and the processed product also has artificial coloring, flavoring and other chemical additives of which most cheese-eaters are not aware.

Most people can easily get used to the taste of foods prepared with little salt, and I am one of those. I think this is one reason why my blood pressure stays low—about 125 over 70. If you have even a slight tendency toward high blood pressure you should make a special effort to eat less salt.

Beverages are often a real health problem in our affluent society. Most tap water tastes bad and is often contaminated with viruses, bacteria, pesticides and chemicals that are not filtered out by treatment plants. Good water is the best of all drinks, but it's getting harder to find with each passing year. People are turning to soft drinks as a favored alternative. The soft drinks whose advertisements promise to make "things go better" for the consumer are largely detrimental to health. This fact is submerged in a blizzard of promotion. True, sales of bottled spring water are rising, but this market is just a drop in the national beverage bucket.

We are fortunate in having our own deep well, which yields a steady supply of pure water. Fresh from the small storage tank, or even out of a garden hose in the summer, it tastes wonderful. Fortunately, it is hard water, because it absorbs desirable minerals as it runs through the limestone strata which underlies our district. People who drink hard water tend to have less heart disease, perhaps because of these minerals, although no one knows exactly why. And of course, it is not fluoridated. Yet all our five children have excellent teeth! Nine-year-old Anthony has no cavities at all. Heidi, now 19, never had a cavity until she was 16.

One more point about water. There are positive health values to be gained from getting yourself into a rather deliberate routine of water-drinking. Some people don't get enough fluids into their bodies. Maybe as we get older our sense of thirst "dries up" to some degree. So while our bodies should actually have more fluid, the thirst mechanism doesn't signal that need often enough. Get around that problem by making a mental note to drink an extra glass of good water every morning and afternoon.

What about alcohol? When I was in my early 20's I got drunk a few times at parties, and for the first ten years or so of married life would pour myself a Scotch and water each evening before dinner. It was the thing to do, I thought. Then gradually I began to realize that the taste of liquor didn't appeal to me (increasingly I found myself pouring away the last half of my drink) and I also noticed that my vitality lagged more after dinner if I had had a drink.

One day it dawned on me that since I didn't like the taste of liquor and enjoyed staying alert, there was really no need to drink at all. It's strange how the obvious is somehow so difficult to see.

My growing involvement with competitive shotgun shooting helped me to make that decision. My hobby of skeet shooting—a clay target game—became almost a passion. For over ten years I have competed in matches all over this country and even in some foreign countries. Drinking and shooting didn't strike me as a good mixture, so I found it no problem at all to stay away from the stuff. Today, I occasionally have white wine with a meal, but I usually drink plain water or club soda at cocktail parties, which I attend infrequently anyway.

Coffee is another drink that I weaned myself from as a result of shooting. As many of you remember, J. I. was a coffee drinker, enjoying its stimulating lift. I found coffee a pleasant drink for many years too, and felt that the extra mental alertness it produces was essential for building up a competitive edge during shooting matches. But while the caffeine in coffee does give you a lift, it is only a temporary one. In nature, there is no action without a reaction, and that applies to the effect of coffee. So during day-long matches I would find myself falling into slump periods when the coffee-effect wore off. Sometimes later in the day, during the difficult final stages of shooting, the snack bar would close and there would be no way to get more coffee. I'd be left to pull myself up by my bootstraps, which is not easy to do.

Gradually, I tapered off until I was drinking only two or three half-cups a day. Then after a few months I stopped drinking coffee entirely. Instead I drank peppermint tea, other herb teas, and sometimes decaffeinated coffee. The effect on my mind and body was quite pronounced. I became much more relaxed, even though I had previously thought of myself as a relaxed person. At first, I suffered from a kind of haziness of the mind, which didn't interfere with my work or thinking, but which was still noticeable. It soon passed, though. My shooting ability suffered for a while, and in fact for a couple of years I lost interest in shooting entirely. But now I am over the hump and feel every bit as clear-headed and energetic as ever.

I am very happy to have kicked the coffee habit. My flow of energy is now much steadier, and I seldom experience the kind of "let down" period that used to be such a problem.

Let's get back to food for a while. You may be curious about how I keep on an organic and natural-food diet while traveling, or when forced to eat in restaurants. That used to be a fairly simple problem. After all, I am not a fanatic about diet and will eat just about any kind of food once or twice, especially to avoid hurting the feelings of a dinner hostess. But the food in restaurants is not as good as it used to be, and it appears to be getting worse. So much restaurant food is now highly processed, instantized, and artifically preserved, colored, and flavored. Even when natural ingredients are used, the quality is not very good. Anyone accustomed to eating organic foods regularly can definitely notice the tremendous difference between that diet and restaurant food.

My technique in a restaurant is to think in terms of eating less. I try to ignore the bread and butter, usually skip the soup (which is often salty and loaded with monosodium glutamate), and avoid dessert unless fresh fruit is available. For a main course I concentrate on fish, chicken or a small piece of meat. I always stay away from complex mixtures and casserole-type foods in restaurants.

Lately, I find myself missing my normal, high-bulk and low fat diet when traveling for long periods. Once you start eating whole grains, cornmeal, beans, nuts and similar foods, you get tuned to that kind of fare—which I think is a very healthful thing. Such foods travel quickly and effortlessly through your system. In my case at least I am never troubled with such typical middle-aged complaints as heartburn and indigestion. When I'm forced to switch away from that kind of diet, the digestive process slows and I get an undefined feeling that somehow all is not well inside.

My remedy is to try to maintain my normal diet as much as possible when traveling. I seek out health food restaurants more often than I used to. Health food stores offer good things that can be eaten while traveling—especially if there is a refrigerator or hot plate in your room. On a recent trip to Australia I bought a big, round loaf of unleavened, whole-grain raisin bread at the Feedwell Food Foundry in Melbourne. It lasted for almost two weeks in my small refrigerator and was especially good as the basic course for breakfast.

Of course, I take food supplements every day—at home or when traveling. I use natural supplements and prefer to take a selection of individual ones rather than rely on an all-in-one product. Here are the food supplements I use:

Bone meal (for calcium and phosphorus)—3 tablets

Dolomite (for magnesium)—3 tablets

Vitamin C with rose hips—from 500 milligrams a day "on up," depending on how I feel and other factors. (More about that later.)

Vitamin E—400 units in 2 capsules

B vitamins—I use a high-B complex formula, and take 3 capsules daily.

Desiccated liver—3 or more tablets.

Vitamin A—25,000 units.

Alfalfa—3 or more tablets a day.

Zinc (from zinc gluconate)—3 tablets, totalling 30 milligrams.

Very often I will add other items to this list, such as kelp tablets, a protein product, or some other natural supplement that is a good source of trace elements. I skip around, to a degree, trying out new things.

Some people measure out all their natural supplements into little bottles, each containing the dosage to be taken before a meal. That method doesn't appeal to me. We keep all the supplement jars on an eye-level shelf in the pantry, and each morning I head there first when I go to the kitchen to make my

23

breakfast. I open each bottle and shake out the tablets or capsules that I want that day. I enjoy sniffing the yeasty smell of the B-vitamin preparation and the hayfield aroma of the alfalfa. Even the bone meal and the vitamin C tablets have distinctive and pleasant aromas, but you'll miss them unless you stick your nose right into the bottle. If the vitamin and mineral tablets were counted out into portion-sized vials for future use, I wouldn't have the chance to do all that smelling.

I also keep vitamin C tablets stashed at several other places—like my briefcase, office desk and bathroom medicine chest. At various times during the day, I'll take a few vitamin C's from these other bottles, especially during cold season, or when I feel a cold or sore throat coming on. I also have a theory that taking a lot of vitamin C makes it easier to jump time zones during long jet flights. I tried it during my recent trip to Australia and got off the plane in Melbourne ready to go, and was soon completely adjusted to the nine-hour time difference.

What other benefits do I get from taking natural supplements? Primarily, I am looking for long-term gains. The chronic, degenerative diseases that strike most people in their mature years—and which even the best medicine is almost powerless to cure completely—are often the result of a life-long marginal intake of vital nutrients like magnesium, calcium, vitamin E and zinc, to name a few. Why not avoid future problems by supplementing the diet now? That is my reasoning, although I feel plenty of current benefits too. Today I am as vigorous, energetic and healthy as ever. In fact I feel much better now than I did when I was in my twenties.

THE SECRET OF FITNESS 3

Without a doubt, becoming physically fit is one of the best—if not *the* best—of all health ideas. The results of a fitness program are quick and dramatic. If you use the right techniques, within a few days you will notice improvement in the shape of your body, increase in your ability to work and to enjoy life's pleasures, better resistance to stress and a more hopeful attitude toward life in general.

The chief stumbling block to initiating and continuing a fitness program is motivation, not weak muscles. So when you consider a fitness program, don't look at your arms and legs, wondering whether you have the strength to go forward—almost everyone has the potential muscle power to improve his fitness in some way. Instead, devote your energies to working out a way to motivate yourself. Try to perfect a strategy for making the necessary muscle-using routines easy and enjoyable. A fitness program must not seem like work to you, or you won't continue it, unless you have tremendous inner resources. Fitness techniques *can* be made enjoyable, or they can become so much a part of your life's routine that you follow them regularly without thinking much about what you are doing.

Closely tied in with the mental aspect of a fitness program—the need for motivation—is the ability to perceive a much larger benefit from fitness than simply improved muscle power. I'm referring to the improvement that it builds into the body's homeostatic mechanisms. Now don't let that word throw you. Just think of it as the body's ability to balance itself internally. You need a sense of balance to stand or walk; you also need balance inside to keep your blood flowing, to keep breathing, and to maintain the proper functioning of all your many glands and organs.

When you allow yourself to become unfit by years of sedentary living, your insides get just as flabby and pudgy as your arms and abdomen. Why? Because some of the most vital inside organs *are* muscles (the heart in particular). If not put under reasonable stress occasionally, they gradually accommodate themselves to an easy life, the same way that your arm and leg muscles weaken and your abdominal muscles droop. And your internal mechanisms also weaken if they are not called upon often enough to counter the challenges that are within the normal range of their activity. For example, when you climb the stairs or use your muscles vigorously in some other way, the muscle cells call out for more glycogen. How well your bloodstream can deliver that extra glycogen depends on whether its "factory" for making and distributing it has been kept "in operation" by frequent exercise.

Your lung efficiency, and even your digestion and elimination systems, are all part of the body's balancing system that is toned up by physical conditioning. When you are unfit, they don't work effectively. The ultimate result is a mental depression that is so common in countries like ours today that it is considered normal. Only those few people who are approaching true fitness know and appreciate the wonderful, clear-headed feeling that an effective homeostatic mechanism produces.

There are plenty of other benefits of a good homeostatic balance, especially in these days of declining energy use. We will have less access to all the technological tricks that make life easier—air conditioning, central heating, escalators—and will have to call upon our own physical resources to adjust to environmental stress. In a heat wave, with no air conditioning, the person with good homeostasis will suffer much less than the unfit person whose internal balance can be thrown off very easily.

Now that you understand the value of homeostasis, you should add this important balance ability to the mental input for your motivation to achieve fitness. In order to get this discussion down to a very practical, how-to-do-it level, I will tell you how I personally have coped with these challenges and have ultimately been able to achieve a fairly good level of fitness for a man with a desk job.

When I was young I put a very low priority on fitness. Although I did a lot of tramping about in the fields and woods, exercise for the sake of self-improvement just didn't interest me. In my early days as an editor I thought that I was destined to be the kind of person who didn't use muscles for much of anything. Then as I got into my thirties, and especially as I became involved in competitive shotgun shooting, my motivation to exercise grew. I realized that since shooting is a physical act as well as a test of mental discipline, a person with overall physical fitness can probably do better. Also, as I read more about health, I became aware of factors like homostasis and also learned how regular, vigorous physical activity might prevent heart disease later in life. I decided that exercise was going to have to become a regular part of my life routine.

Running was the central part of my first exercise plan. I started jogging around the fields in back of my house. I enjoyed running and soon increased my distance to the point where I was covering four or five miles a day, on nearby country roads. Then trouble struck! A ligament injury in my left leg caused me pain. Instead of training gradually, working up slowly to vigorous running, I had strained for improvement and seriously injured myself. For a while, my exercise program had to stop.

Some authorities say it is inevitable that runners and even joggers will injure themselves at some time or another. They are probably right, but that is no reason to avoid exercise entirely. Fitness is so valuable that it is worth pursuing even at the risk of possible shin splints and tendonitis. Remember, if you have been sedentary for ten or more years, your muscles and especially ligaments are probably in very weak condition. You need to work slowly and gently until they are gradually strengthened. Take precautions to protect yourself. Train, don't strain. If you do that, you have little to fear from injury.

My next exercise phase was calisthenics. The Royal Canadian Air Force calisthenic program was then popular, as was a routine put out by the President's Council on Physical Fitness. I tried the President's Council program for five or six months, but found that a greater and greater mental effort was needed each day to continue. Finally, thoroughly bored, I gave up.

There I was, without an exercise program to call my own. But the need and the motivation to exercise still existed. Every month, through my reading I learned more about how vital good physical condition is to the enjoyment of life. I also had an important personal goal of qualifying for membership on the 1968 U. S. Olympic Team in my specialty of international skeet shooting.

I discovered that the distance between my home and office was ideal for a good walk—2.8 miles. Walking to work and back each day would be a perfect way to get in shape! But as you might surmise, it took quite a mental adjustment, and also some physical conditioning, to make the switch from being a driving commuter to being a walker.

Simple questions had to be answered, but they nevertheless required planning. What would I wear? What would I do if it started raining half way to work? How would I carry the journals and papers which I usually bring home to read at night? The need to work these things out indicated how dependent I had become on the mechanical contrivances of our technological society.

After considerable preparation—equipped with hiking boots, a bright orange coat easily seen by cars, and a canvas shoulder bag for my papers—I set out on that first walk. Forty-five minutes later, perspired and tired, I reached the office, feeling as if I had completed a minor expedition. Late that afternoon I dragged myself home by the same route.

Now I walk to work quite regularly, sometimes five days a week. And looking back over my experience as a walking commuter, what comes to mind most clearly is the remarkable improvement in walking stamina that I have achieved—that improvement has come slowly and steadily over a period of at least two years.

After only a few weeks of doing without the car as much as possible, I was able to walk to work and back without any strain at all. But then I tried some longer distances—say seven or eight miles—and found the effort quite taxing. But after a year of walking 2.8 miles to work and back, I found that I could walk ten or even 15 miles in a few hours and not feel any strain at all. Sometimes I made those long walks with a 30-pound pack on my back, too, and the extra weight didn't bother me.

So keep in mind that if you have led a sedentary life, you probably will have to train yourself gradually in order to make long walks happy affairs. But you can look forward to steady improvement in your walking strength if you persist in a walking program for several years.

Another gain from walking is mental peace and calmness. At first when you start walking you will miss having that car radio to listen to, and perhaps you will also be in a rather big hurry to get where you're going. As a matter of fact, I found my first several walks quite boring, but as the months passed my mind shifted gears. The peacefulness of that 45-minute interlude each morning and evening became something to treasure and look forward to. The boredom was replaced by meditation, and now when I have to drive because of bad weather, or when I need the car for work, I find myself unhappy about missing my walk.

Occasionally I use a bicycle for the trip to work, especially in the summer. Riding a 10-speed bike provides almost as much exercise, per mile, covered as walking (if you have a few good hills to go up, as I do), and it offers the chance for a change of pace. Using the bike also cuts a half-hour off my commuting time.

In addition, cycling exercises different muscles than walking, an advantage to anyone searching for total fitness. Most important, though, the bicycle has opened up a whole new world of activity and fitness interest to me. There's nothing to beat the unique sense of mobility-under-your-own-power that long bicycle rides can give.

On weekends, I will take off for 20 to 40 miles

through the pleasant Pennsylvania back country around Allentown. Quietly wheeling along with the wind whispering in my ears, I sneak up on cows in their pastures and ducks in their marshes. Usually I head west, against the prevailing winds, then cycle easily home with the breeze pushing me along. The greatest fun of all is to ride home with a very strong wind at my back, with my speed matching that of the wind exactly. The road moves quickly beneath the wheels, yet I feel as if I am riding in still air. It is almost like being weightless in space.

Bicycling is bound to increase in popularity. Not only is it fun, but cycling is the most energy-efficient of all methods of human transportation. You can get farther on fewer calories with a bicycle than in any other way, including walking. That's why the Chinese use many millions of bicycles, as do Europeans, Asians and Africans. Wherever there is a need for cheap transportation, and where gasoline is either expensive or not available, the bicycle is king.

You may think that cycling is not exactly your cup of tea. But soon more people of all ages, sizes, and states of physical condition will be trying bicycling, so why not try your hand at it? My suggestion is that you give very strong consideration to the 10-speed type of bicycle, with the turned-down handlebars. Riding that kind of bike isn't as uncomfortable as it looks, and in fact is quite pleasant once you get used to it. Just remember that starting slowly is important. You may need months of short trips before your legs and ligaments build up the strength you need to power you on long bicycle journeys.

By way of summing up, here are the two best ideas about fitness that I have learned:

1. Much more benefit can be gained from spending a lot of time at gentle exercise than from rushing through a vigorous workout. I found, for

example, that after a year of walking to work, my pulse rate lowered considerably and my lung-power increased, even though I never got out of breath or felt that I was doing any really vigorous exercise. What did the trick was the fact that I was spending an hour and a half a day at some form of exercise—even though it was mild exercise.

Too many people think of exercise as something best done in a few minutes (or even seconds) a day. Of course, any reasonable exercise is better than none, but I believe that fitness is much *easier* to achieve when you decide to do gentle things like walking and cycling for as long a time each day as possible. You can then motivate yourself to exercise more easily, because gentle, rhythmic activity is both relaxing and fun. And if you do it outdoors you entertain yourself easily by having a constant change of scenery.

Walking or cycling is an escape from the cares of the day, while the five-minute calisthenic routine is a constraint, another rigid requirement of the rat-race kind of life. In fact, I find it easier to get in the habit of using more than an hour to day to walk back and forth to work, than to force myself to take a couple of minutes to do push-ups or knee-bends. And I get much more benefit from the longer exercise session.

2. Getting warmed up slowly and completely is crucial to appreciating the strength that is in your own body—even if you lack fitness. Warming up is almost equivalent to "starting your engine," if, for a moment, you think of your body as a car. The strength is there, but it isn't ready for efficient use until you start the juices flowing.

Most people who don't do any physical work never experience the joy and power of that warmed-up feeling. That's a shame, because they are underestimating their physical potential. Once you are warmed up, you have the feeling that your body was made to move, and to keep moving.

The best way to describe the warmed-up feeling is to tell what happens to me when I get on my bicycle. For the first few blocks—or even longer, if the weather is cold—my legs feel heavy and unresponsive. Pedaling seems more like work than fun. But then after the perspiration pops out I gradually get the feeling that I can keep going on and on—with much less effort. My mental outlook changes, too. I become much happier about being on a bicycle after I push through the barrier of "coldness."

Some experts feel that being warmed-up properly not only makes the effort easier, but also protects against muscle injury. How do you get warmed up? The best way is to put on what the athletes call a warm-up suit, and just start moving about gently. Walk, jog a little, shake your arms and kick your legs. Alternate walking with jogging, but take your time. Gradually, perhaps after ten or 15 minutes, you get the feeling that your body is more alive, and ready to take on new challenges. Then you're warmed up, you're really ready to get moving!

FOODS AND HERBS IN FOLK MEDICINE 4

Call it folklore—or folk medicine—or whatever you will. There's still no getting around the fact that our grandfathers and their fathers before them knew a great deal about practical things that science has since attempted to discard.

They knew about health—which herbal remedy to take if you were coming down with a cold or fighting an infection from injury or disease. They knew about the natural world—the everturning seasons, the changing heavens above their heads, when to plant seeds for best results.

Our grandfathers knew all those things, but little by little, in our fathers' lifetimes and in ours, most of this knowledge was lost, forsaken for the new and "better" ways of technology, mass production and mass marketing. Now, however, scientists are independently rediscovering much of the truth behind the old lore. And they are finding that the old, natural ways really are the best ways.

For example, is getting to sleep a problem for you? If so, you may be interested to know that English scientists have now proven the old belief that a drink of warm milk before bedtime can literally "knock you out" and give you a good night's rest.

The work was done at Royal Edinburgh Hospital and Guy's Hospital Medical School in London, and was reported in the *British Medical Journal* (May 20, 1972). Remarkably, the effect of the bedtime drink was most significant toward morning, when sleep usually becomes lighter and more fitful. And the effect of the drink grew stronger with continued use. That's just the opposite of commercial sleep-inducing drugs, whose effects taper off, leading you to take ever-larger doses.

Another food-related goal of many people is regular bowel movements. Judging from sales of laxatives, America is a nation of constipation sufferers. Some people go through life using these drugs as a crutch, debilitating the power of their intestines to act in normal ways.

Curing constipation with food is the simplest and most natural of such treatments, provided you know what to eat and are willing to avoid the foods that are causing your problem.

Cut out white flour and sugared, refined foods for a start. They have long been known as contributors to irregularity, because of their lack of fiber and bulk. Substitute whole grain and unrefined cereal products. Don't fret about the "different" taste of those foods. Stick with them and you'll soon think they taste great.

Other classic anti-constipation foods include raisins, prunes, figs, salads, and unpeeled apples. High-cellulose foods like tomatoes, cantaloupes, peas and beans provide fibrous bulk in the lower intestine. Tough foods like nuts and seeds also help keep bowel function regular.

Adequate bulk and fiber in your diet can do more than just prevent constipation. There is ample evidence that it can prevent diseases of the bowel—diverticulosis, appendicitis and even cancer of the colon.

Africans and other primitive people rarely get any of these diseases because of the large amount of unabsorbable fiber they consume every day, Dr. Denis P. Burkitt recently reported to an audience at the University of Iowa. When grains are not refined to "naked starch" by modern milling techniques, "you are totally free of all noninfective disease of the bowel," said this Englishman who has spent years studying the health of the rural African.

"We have assumed that we can take the unabsorbable fiber from our food and it doesn't matter because we say it's got no nourishment," Dr. Burkitt said. Our forefathers, of course, never made such an erroneous assumption. They let nature dictate their diet. And nature's fruits, vegetables and whole grain provided all the fibrous material their systems needed.

Calmness and peace of mind are other qualities that many people are now seeking through diet change. The boom in the study of Eastern cultures—like yoga—that promise new insights into life, also reflects the belief that a return to a more natural diet is important to the way you think and feel.

Up to now, little research has been done on the effect of food on mental attitudes, because no organization with sufficient money is interested in the question.

But one indication of just how dramatically food can alter our mental attitudes is provided by George Watson, Ph.D., in his book *Nutrition and Your Mind* (Harper & Row, 1972). When some thirty male volunteers were placed on a semistarvation diet, Dr. Watson relates, "the group as a whole showed marked personality changes, both neurotic and psychotic. In fact, some subjects became so disturbed that they inflicted physical damage on themselves. One of the conclusions offered by the scientists who did this research was that 'experimental neurosis' could be induced entirely by nutritional means.''

One definite way to change your mental outlook with diet—is to stop drinking coffee. Caffeine is a powerful stimulant and can change the way you think and act. Stopping coffee suddenly will slow down your pace of life, but for many people that's desirable in these hectic times.

Our forefathers drank many delicious hot beverages made from herbs of various sorts. These drinks did a great deal more good than coffee, and what's more, they didn't need sugar to make them palatable.

Non-coffee drinkers are frequently fans of herbal teas (also called tisanes) which have been known for centuries to possess mildly medicinal and psychological effects. Some of the most popular herb teas are camomile, catnip, mint and sassafras. Most often they are served warm, but can be used for iced tea also.

Reviving Interest in the Antique Foods

Maybe you can get a better picture of how our grandfathers approached diet and food selection by traveling back in time, at least in your imagination. A trip around America used to lead to many regional food adventures. You discovered unique country hams in the South, ocean-fresh lobster in New England, and tasty steaks in Kansas City.

Today, you usually have to settle for feed-lot beef everywhere. It's tender, but fatty and bland in flavor. And from Maine to California, your breakfast eggs are graced by dehydrated potato shreds.

The regional specialties are still there, of course,

but they've been largely smothered by a flood of standardized food, homogenized in vast factories to cater to the average palate. Gone are the constant flavor surprises of years ago.

Growing your own food is a good way to get nutritious foods with a different flavor. Every September literally millions of people are busy canning, freezing and drying produce from their gardens and homesteads. There's also interest in reviving what I call "antique" foods, like dried string beans ("leather britches") and real homemade sauerkraut.

Some of the old-time foods have become popular enough to be available in supermarkets, and others stayed popular through the period when convenience foods were thought to be the be-all and end-all of good eating. Usually, you'll find the specialties of your own region in local markets.

Foods making a comeback all over the country include whole grains, water ground cornmeal, and brown rice. They have the advantage of being relatively inexpensive and can combine with other foods to add interest and variety to almost any menu.

Natural cheeses are also growing in popularity. They are not homogenized, processed or preserved, so they don't last indefinitely without refrigeration. But in exchange for that convenience you get the rustic taste of what all cheese was like years ago. The longer you keep them in the refrigerator, the stronger their flavor gets.

Strongly smoked, home-cured meats are also arousing the interest of people looking for unusual flavors, but I advise approaching them with caution. The rate of stomach cancer in the U. S. has been declining, and some experts theorize that the reason is lower consumption of smoked meats. There is evidence that smoked foods are cancer-causing if eaten to excess.

Plenty of safe, healthful old-time foods are available for people who take the time to look around. Roadside stands sometimes offer things like Jerusalem artichokes, in season. They're tubers of a sunflower-like plant and are excellent when served raw in salads.

If you have a chance to find hickory nuts, either whole or shelled, snap them up. Although not commercialized like black walnuts, they are the best nuts for adding to baked goods.

A special treat that our ancestors scoured the woods to find was early spring asparagus. Not only is this wild vegetable tender and delicious, its high vitamin content makes it especially valuable.

I think you'll agree our forefathers had the right idea about what good eating, and good health, is all about.

The Chinese System of Herbal Medicine

The Chinese also have some "right ideas" about good health. The use of Chinese herbs is a fascinating subject full of questions, and your very first question might be—why *Chinese* herbs? Every country has its own armamentarium of herbal drugs. We can find plenty of plant drug resources in the health culture of the American Indians, the Spanish settlers of our Southwest, or among the descendants of the English, Scotch and Irish pioneers who homesteaded the Appalachia.

The answer is that we could use herbs from anywhere, but our goal should not be just to use herbs. It should be to build with herbs in a positive way, and to do that we have to be certain that the traditional health culture we are dipping into has the highest possible percentage of validity, effectiveness, and real health-improving value.

No part of the world has contributed more valuable plants to our culture than China. Its flora is remarkably diverse and useful.

In population too, China is out in front. Her land area has supported hundreds of millions of people for many generations. The great misfortunes that the Chinese people have experienced—countless epidemics, earthquakes, floods and famines—have forced her people to use literally every plant that grows in that country, as food or drug. Nowhere else on earth has there ever been such a large "laboratory" for the development of herbal medicines as in China.

Herbal Drug Stores

On my recent trip to the People's Republic of China, I found that the use of herbs and natural drugs was a routine part of life for the majority of people. True, antibiotics and synthetic drugs of various types are available and are used, but herbal drugs appear to be much more common. For example, you can walk down Nanking Road, the main shopping street of Shanghai, now the world's most populous city, and find many more herb medicine shops than conventional drug stores. Even the stores selling synthetic medicines have a small herb department.

The sale of herbal drugs in stores is only one part of the picture. All Chinese people are encouraged to take some responsibility for the collection of materials used to make natural medicines. For example, signs in the little neighborhood offices of part-time health workers ask people to save tangerine peels, cuttlefish shells, and other items so that they can be "recycled" as ingredients in natural drugs. Each regiment of the army has a garden of as many as 500 different types of medicinal plants. The soldiers are taught to identify all those plants so that while on maneuvers they can collect the raw materials for natural drugs. The medical unit of the regiment has a small pharmaceutical factory which converts the raw plants into useful medications.

Actually, the 500 types of medicinal plants grown in an army herb garden are only a fraction of the natural medicines used in China. The average herb shop carries a selection of 2,000 different items, and the Chinese claim that an additional 1,000 plants, useful for medical purposes, were discovered during the Cultural Revolution. Those new plants are now being tested more thoroughly. A variety of herbal reference books is published in China. Many have color illustrations with the plants identified by their Latin names as well as Chinese characters. Each province of China, in fact, publishes its own herbal guide, because there is great variation in the types of native plants available for medicinal use in different regions.

The large variety of plants used as health promoters in China brings us face to face with the question of how we, as alien Westerners, can make use of this vast health resource. It is not an easy question to answer. While in Shanghai, I spent almost half an hour chatting, through an interpreter, with a pharmacist in a large herb shop on Nanking Road. My basic question was this: "Of the 2,000 different natural medicines you stock, which are the best sellers?" I asked for a list of the 10 most popular items, so that I could come back home and write a simple, easily understood article giving Americans some clue as to where to start using Chinese natural medicine.

I got nowhere with this fellow, although he was

trying to cooperate. Finally, I understood what he was endeavoring to tell me. There are no best-selling Chinese herbs—all 2,000 are used regularly by large numbers of people. Why should that be? My first thought was that, since there is no advertising of any products in China, the state-owned companies marketing herbal products don't have a chance to promote 5 or 6 favorite items heavily—the way Anacin or Alka-Seltzer are pushed here.

Later I realized that there is a much more important reason for the wide use of such a large number of different herbs. The Chinese people are taught how to collect, compound and use herbal products from childhood. Such natural medications are a part of the very fabric of their lives. The average person has a large reservoir of herb lore. And in addition, the Chinese often use more than one herb at a time. They get prescriptions that are made up from perhaps a dozen or more different plants, parts of birds and animals, and other things from nature. It is little wonder that a store clerk can be kept busy dipping into 2,000 different bins and drawers.

The large number of plants used by the Chinese should not be a barrier to our use of their herb culture. Just the opposite! Such variety is the best evidence we can get of the richness of Chinese herb lore.

The Chinese are developing simpler ways for their herbal products to be used by people who were not brought up in an herb-using society.

The Techniques of Herbalism

Before becoming too enmeshed in specific Chinese ideas about herbs, let's consider two broader questions. First, why should we be interested in herbs at all? And second, how can we make a start toward meeting our health goals with herbs?

43

The simple answer to the first question is that herbs are natural and therefore largely-safe, health-building and curative agents. We are badly in need of such safety. Every day new synthetic compounds are introduced into our environment, without anyone knowing what their long-range effect will be. Many of those artificial chemicals are drugs, and we have been able to document that most can have very harmful effects, especially when misused.

The synthetic drug usually operates by unbalancing one of the body's normal systems to correct a specific symptomatic problem. There are side effects, sometimes quite serious, especially when two or more such drugs are used together or in conjunction with alcohol or environmental contaminants. When you realize that many people use drugs every day, or even every few hours, you begin to understand just how big the drug-side-effects problem is. Very often, the original illness is replaced by one or more other, and sometimes more serious, problems that are in reality side effects. It is a vicious cycle that traps millions of people.

Herbal preparations offer a way out of this drug trap. Consider camomile tea, for example. It is known to contain substances which have a mild calming and tranquilizing effect. The Chinese use it, as well as people from many other countries. One cup will not put you into never-never land, like a Librium tablet, but if you drink camomile tea regularly several times a day, you will gradually note that it makes you feel more relaxed. If more people would take the camomile tea route to the solution of problems of sleeplessness or mild anxiety, we would have a much healthier society—and probably could save money in the process.

Let's consider my second question—how can we make a start toward meeting our health goals with herbs more effectively? Frankly, I don't think that's going to be very hard to do. True, using herbs for health would be easier if we had a million herb doctors to guide us, the way the Chinese do, and if we had herb stores on every street. But even without those resources, there are ways to use more health herbs in our lives.

After all, many of these medicinal plants are as common as weeds in our gardens. Some of them actually *are* weeds! Unless you live in a high-rise city apartment, chances are that there are some useful wild plants now growing within a few hundred feet of where you are now sitting. A barefoot-doctors' herbal that I brought back from China lists dandelion, plantain and a host of other very common plants as useful for a variety of health purposes.

Treatment for a Cold— Chinese Style

My opportunity to try real Chinese herbs, administered by a Chinese doctor, presented itself while I was in Shanghai. No one hopes to get sick, but when my throat began to thicken-up one day I thought, "Here's my chance to learn about the Chinese medical system at first hand." Our hosts would cooperate, of course. All five of the guides and interpreters for our group were continually solicitous of our health, and had a doctor in our room at the first sign of a sniffle or stomachache.

My desire was to get just a little bit sick so I could go to a traditional Chinese doctor and see how he would treat me. As you may know, the traditional system of medicine in China is based on almost entirely different principles than Western medicine. Herbal medicine, more commonly called traditional medicine, is a trial-and-error thing that has evolved over thousands of years. People got sick and took various herbs, fungi, animal bones—alone or in combination—and waited to see if they got better.

Because it wasn't scientific, Chinese traditional medicine was put in a secondary position by the communist government for quite a few years. Herbal medicine didn't appear to be the wave of the future, but then the country people of China had no alternative to such simple methods. Herbs and acupuncture were the only things they had to keep them healthy.

Acupuncture had evolved the same way—stick yourself with needles to see if that persistent rheumatism or arthritis pain goes away. There was very little basic research or even science connected with the development of Chinese traditional medicine. All that counted was getting better—not why you got better.

Of course, there are weaknesses to Chinese traditional medicine. It isn't as effective as Western medicine in some areas, where our science has opened up new vistas of the working of the human body. The Chinese realize that, and in their inherently wise way they are combining the two systems. All doctors in China today must know at least something about both methods of treatment. Chairman Mao decreed the merger of Western and traditional medicine during the Cultural Revolution, and the herb "business" in China has been booming ever since.

Back to my sore throat. Getting a cold in North China in January is ridiculously easy, even for a vitamin C fan, like me. The buildings are either overheated, unheated, or slightly-warmed by tiny soft-coal stoves or charcoal braziers.

My herb doctor, Dr. Sheng Lui-Chi, was a kindly, relaxed gentleman of 73 years. Dressed in a white lab coat, he looked superficially like a Western doctor, but his manner was far different. Dr. Sheng did not rush me through the clinic so he could get to the next patient. He seemed to almost draw a shell around himself so he could think my case through while feeling my pulse for several minutes at a time —first on one wrist and then the other, using three fingers to sense the rhythm and pressure of the beats.

He asked me a few questions: "What bothers you? Is your mouth dry? Do you feel hot and perspired?"

Of course, the questioning was in Chinese and the answers were supplied through Mr. Yang Shan-Hou, my interpreter. Dr. Sheng didn't examine my chest with a stethoscope, although he did glance at my throat. His diagnosis appeared to be mainly pulse-oriented, with his fingers changing their pressure on my wrist from time to time, seeking some information which was completely unfathomable to me.

After completing his written diagnosis, Dr. Sheng explained my treatment program to Mr. Yang, who passed the details along to me. The cold was to be treated with two medications. First, there were some pills. "Take 10 before each meal," I was told.

"Ten pills at a time!" That's a lot, I mused as I put the little drug envelope in my pocket without looking at its contents.

Then there was the herb medicine. Dr. Sheng explained that the medicine he preferred to use in my case would require cooking, and perhaps some traditional Chinese folk wisdom about the use of herb medicines which I obviously didn't possess. So he said he was compromising by giving me an herb blend that I could steep in the big, covered tea cup which is a fixture of all Chinese hotel rooms. Dr. Sheng also gave me a supply of gauze pieces with which to filter out the "grounds" after 15 minutes of immersion. "Drink it twice a day," he said, "and you can use the mixture a second time, just by adding water to it again."

My questioning of Dr. Sheng was very brief, because he had already given me more of his valuable time than my simple upper respiratory infection—which was less than a day old—justified. I established only that he was trained in Western medicine to a certain extent, but was predominantly a traditional herb doctor. His large, bright, impressive clinic and waiting room at the East China Hospital in Shanghai testified to the importance of his professional position.

Then came a surprise. One of the nice women who had been hovering in the background, gossiping about either me or the treatment I was getting, turned out to be Dr. Yo Chi-Wei, an acupuncture specialist.

"Would you like me to treat your cold with acupuncture?" she asked.

"Of course," I replied.

She pointed to the adjoining room with a hospital bed and invited me to take off my shoes and jacket and sit on the bed. The preliminary lecture was extremely brief.

"You will feel only a small prick when the needle goes in," Dr. Yo told me, "Don't be afraid. There may be a slight numbness, which is a sign that the treatment is working."

Thus prepared, I awaited the first insertions, which came in the back of the neck, at what felt to me to be the base of my hairline. They were noticeable pricks, not exactly pleasant but not as annoying as the jab of a hypodermic needle. And the needles remained in for only a few seconds.

"Why did you put the needles there?" I asked.

"Because your cold comes partly from wind striking the back of your neck," she replied.

I couldn't argue with that logic, and awaited her next effort. It came in the form of a needle in each hand, in the fleshy part between thumb and forefinger.

"These two needles will stay in for ten minutes," Dr. Yo informed me.

They didn't feel like much going in, and I rested quite comfortably for about five minutes. Then I began to feel like the needle in my right hand was causing something significant to happen to my body. It didn't hurt, but my hand and even my arm got slightly numb. I can only describe it as a kind of "flowing numbness," which I called to the attention of Dr. Yo.

"That means the treatment is working," she replied. "You may even feel something for a few hours after the needles are removed."

I waited, with the sensation increasing, and as she removed that needle from my right hand I felt a blast of the kind of energy that acupuncture can produce. My whole right side was terrifically stimulated for an instant. It was not exactly a feeling of pain, nor of an electric shock, but what I can best describe as a blast of concentrated energy.

By that time, I had been at the East China Hospital for over an hour. I had been exposed to quite a bit of Chinese traditional medicine but I didn't have to pay any bill. The twenty-three dollars-a-day we had paid to China Travel Service for our trip covered everything—room, meals, laundry, train and plane tickets, haircuts—even hospitalization, if necessary.

That afternoon I prepared a brew from one of my four packets of mixed herbs. It turned out to be dark and rich in appearance—like the strongest of coffees. I can only describe the flavor as not unpleasant, yet not exactly pleasant either—just overwhelmingly medicinal.

The pills, of which I was to take ten before each meal, gave me a laugh. They were so small, almost invisible without a magnifying glass. Counting out ten took me at least fifteen minutes—constantly shifting pills back and forth from the tiny vial to a dish. But I managed to separate roughly ten from the main supply.

The next day my throat was worse and I couldn't speak at all. Our group left very early for Hangchow, and I spent the three-hour trip conserving my vocal cords. Even under the best of circumstances, little better was to be expected. My cold was less than a day old when I consulted Dr. Sheng and Dr. Yo, and quite frankly I didn't expect their treatment to work miracles. My purpose in seeing them was primarily to "get a handle" on Chinese medicine, and my cold was really just the agent for doing that.

Noticing my discomfort, our Hangchow hosts again called in a doctor, a charming young lady named Sung Kuang Tsao. She showed up with a plastic flight bag packed with medicines in one hand and a yellow flashlight in the other. Dr. Sung took my temperature in the armpit—the Chinese way. The temperature was normal—36.6 degrees Centigrade. She then examined my throat briefly, noted the extent of its infection, and told me to eat oranges, drink plenty of water, and avoid hot, spicy foods for a few days.

She also left me a new medicine, stranger than anything I had yet seen. It was a small, brown, olive-like object which she told me to steep in boiling water for fifteen minutes, then drink the liquid. The name of this traditional drug was *Pon Tai Hai*. I found out later that it's a seed from an Indonesian shrub.

Soon after being placed in the hot water, the little nut sent out filaments and in a quarter of an hour expanded into a brown jellyfish-like thing—not at all appetizing to look at. The broth tasted O.K.—although it didn't have quite the superlative medicinal flavor of Dr. Sheng's prescription, which was a mixture of many herbs.

I didn't want to put Dr. Sung on the spot by inquiring too deeply into her medical background. But my guess is that she is well under 30 and is not trained as completely as our doctors.

Be that as it may, the next day my cold was much better and was almost completely gone the day following. Of course, I had continued to take vitamin C, but even with vitamins, my colds—which I get about once a year—usually last a week and sometimes even longer. To shake one in three days is something new for me—and a tribute to the effectiveness of Chinese traditional medicine.

What a Garden Can Be

We can learn from the wisdom of the Chinese and look to the land for more of our answers.

A garden doesn't have to be just a garden. It can also be a source of unique and sometimes mystical (because we don't understand them) properties that help us live longer, look better, feel better and save plenty of money while doing all three.

Diversity of species is what makes plants so useful to us for health-building purposes. Grasses, trees, vines, shrubs, herbs, and legumes of almost infinite types cover our land, each with a distinctive and different chemical pattern in its cells. They taste different, smell different to us and to insects, and have varying effects when eaten. And in some of those unique plant cells are potent healing sub-

51

stances. A plant that may seem entirely useless as food or for any other purpose can have in its tissue the power to prevent or control serious human illness.

Our lands are now covered by almost endless fields of corn, beans and grains, all of similar hybrid type. Once those fields were full of plant types as different as the people you could see walking down a busy street. Corn was not all of the same cytoplasm, as it is likely to be today, but varied from plant to plant. Weeds between the plants could not be completely controlled, because those potent, weed-killing chemicals hadn't come along yet.

Weeds! There's an interesting concept for you. The very word weed smacks of a totally useless, damaging and insidiously harmful plant. The idea that any plant can be completely bad is relatively new, created by the dollar hungry farmers who are squeezed economically into making every inch of their land pay off at the bank. Old-time country people didn't always like weeds, of course, but they knew how to use many of those derelict plants in time of need. There was a feeling of kinship toward everything in the plant world. Dandelion was not a pest, but a source of salad greens in the spring and winemakings in the summer. No matter how hard you worked during the day to chop a weed from the cotton, you might wish you had a sprig or two later for flavoring, to make tea, or to cure some ailment.

Plant medicine is not always completely effective or safe, of course. People who used oil of sassafras to cure syphilis, as they did for several hundred years, didn't get better unless they were among the thirty percent who got better spontaneously. And plants can be poisonous, as with poison ivy, poison hemlock and many others. Chemicals from plant cells are potent, sometimes even more so than their synthetic chemical copies. But through trial and error people have learned which plants to avoid for certain purposes, and have passed that information along to their children so they'd not make damaging mistakes. Considering the big gaps in our knowledge of health and disease that used to exist—and still do —plants have served extremely well as a source of drugs, food supplements, and general health-builders over the centuries.

The pendulum has now swung the other way. Thanks to chemistry, modern scientists are interested in plants mainly to find pharmaceutical material that they can copy cheaply in laboratories. Crews of pharmacognosists (strange word, meaning an expert on using plants for health) still roam the wilds looking for plant tissue that can be useful in making drugs. But their finds reach the market as a chemical reflection of what was in the natural plant, a copy made synthetically in the lab. It's too expensive these days to collect or cultivate plants for health, except in a few instances. We are living in an increasingly synthetic age.

Clearly, it is time to focus our attention once more on the health-giving power of plants, without turning away entirely from modern medicines. And just as I would not urge you to avoid all synthetic medicines, especially in time of dire need, I do urge you to look at the health-producing power of plants in a creative, selective way, for plants are far from being all good. I am not impressed by arguments that psychedelic drugs made from plants are natural, therefore are acceptable to everyone.

Folklore of Plant Medicine

Examples of Plants and Uses:
Below are examples of how our ancestors used flowers, herbs and seeds.

FLOWERS

Chrysanthemum—Good to combine with camomile flowers. Used for fever.

Cloves—Increase circulation, promote digestion, relieve gastric and intestinal pains.

Lavender—Headache, vomiting, hemorrhages, paralysis.

Marigolds—Abscesses, ulcers, vomiting.

HERBS

Hoarhound—Gastric ulcer, constipation, hepatitis, jaundice, inflammations.

Hyssop—Bronchial asthma, tonsillitis, trachoma.

Marshmallow—Pneumonia, tonsillitis, toothache.

Nettle—Heart disease, gout, obesity, inflammations, laryngitis, fevers.

Peppermint Leaves—Gastritis, vomiting, influenza, headache, toothaches.

Rosemary Leaves—Heart disease, gastritis, diarrhea, obesity.

Sage—Vertigo, wound infections.

SEEDS

Fennel—Constipation, colic, coughs, convulsions, cramps, fevers.

Fenugreek—Ulcers, pneumonia, asthma, rheumatism, abscesses, tumors, laryngitis.

Mustard—Dyspepsia, hyperacidity, gout, intoxication.

ROOTS

Comfrey—(whole plant can be used) Ulcers, sores, tumors.

Hellebore (Black-Root)—Respiratory and heart trouble.

Licorice—Chronic constipation, gallstones, pneumonia, pleurisy.

May-Apple—Liver troubles.

Musk—Gastric insufficiency, dyspepsia, bronchial asthma, fevers.

TREES (BARK, LEAVES, ETC.)

American Boxwood—Bark of root when dried used for fevers; fruit for stomach disorders; twigs used for tooth powder.

Chinese Cinnamon Bark—Gastritis, diarrhea, toothache, fevers.

Eucalyptus Leaves—Gastritis, bronchial asthma, malaria, toothache.

Hemlock (Water-Bark)—Retention of urine, coughs, heachache, fevers.

Horse Chestnut—Bark, seeds and fruit used for hemorrhoids, stimulating nerves; bark solution for fever; outside application for ulcers.

Juniper Berries and Twigs—Vomiting, coughs, treated with twigs. Berries used for hepatitis, gallstones, jaundice, pneumonia, obesity, paralysis, hysteria and cramps.

Oak Bark—Nose bleeds, gastric disorders, ulcers.

Slippery Elm—Inner bark used to heal all kinds of wounds, allay coughs, sore throat, inflammation.

WEEDS

Dandelion leaves and Roots—Diarrhea, chronic constipation, fevers.

Honeysuckle—Asthma and lung trouble; will relieve bee sting.

OTHER PLANTS

Aloe Vera—Juice from leaves good for wounds and burns of all kinds.

Blackberry—Leaves and roots used as astringent medicine for children; also for dysentery and diarrhea.

Hawthorn Berry—Mildly dilates coronary blood vessels; used for "degenerative" heart conditions, narrowing of the arteries, etc.

Hops—Insomnia, abscesses, ulcers, fevers.

Rhubarb—Anemia, gastritis, chronic constipation.

Sphagnum Moss—Dressing wounds. Gather whole, squeeze, dry in air.

Strawberry Leaves—Cases of retention of urine, lowered vitality.

Watercress—Heart disease.

Garlic—A Plant That Deserves Consideration

If you are going to use plants to try to improve your health, you must be willing to seek out facts for yourself. Information about the health-building power of plants is available from many books and articles, but it is not so readily obtained from doctors or other medical practitioners. Most of them are still too indoctrinated in the use of commercial drugs, and too uneducated in plant and herbal lore.

One plant that deserves serious consideration for its curative power is garlic. It has long been a standby of folk medicine practitioners and has been widely used over the centuries to treat hot flashes, flu, head colds, high blood pressure, indigestion and infections. And that's not by any means a complete list of the things that garlic is reported to do.

Whenever a plant or drug is said to have so many different values, people tend to become skeptical. But the strange thing about garlic is that objective testing shows that it really does work, at least for most of those problems if not all of them. Doctor F. G. Piotrowsky of the University of Geneva found in 1948 that garlic helps lower blood pressure by opening up tight blood vessels. And by doing that, garlic also bring relief from dizziness, angina pains and headaches.

Despite such findings, a plant like garlic is not likely to become popular with modern physicians because it is not as high-powered a remedy as many of the new synthetic drugs. For example, high blood pressure is a more common disease today than it was a generation ago, and doctors want drugs that will knock it down more effectively than a gentle, natural remedy can. But that shouldn't stop people from using garlic on their own, either in its food form or as food supplements, which are available without the usual garlic smell. There will be no harmful side effects, and the evidence of garlic's value is sufficiently convincing to justify its use.

Of particular interest is the possibility that garlic grown organically may have much more potency than garlic grown in soil treated with chemical fertilizers. This finding was recently reported by David L. Greenstock after eight years of research conducted on behalf of the Henry Doubleday Research Association in England. He discovered that an oil of garlic emulsion used as an insecticide killed eighty-nine percent of aphids and ninety-five percent of onion flies. But for garlic to have this effect, according to Greenstock, it was necessary that the plants be able to take up certain essential nutrients from the soil, and that called for the presence of ample soil microorganisms and fungi. Ideal conditions for growing garlic with proper potency were found only in an organically treated soil.

Ginseng—Easy to be Suspicious About

Another plant which deserves special mention is ginseng. This is an easy plant to be suspicious about. The Chinese have used extracts of ginseng root for a thousand years or more as a general tonic, curative, strength-builder and aphrodisiac. But until recently, there has been no evidence, of a scientific character, that ginseng really does what the Chinese say it does. What turned me off for a long time was the well-known story that the Chinese place extremely high value on ginseng roots that are shaped in the form of a human being, with a fat trunk and root branches that look like arms and legs. What better evidence could there be that ginseng is some kind of voodoo plant, not a legitimate medicinal herb?

For a long time, I lived a completely ginseng-free life, skeptical of the stories that it makes you feel good again in some mysterious way. Then one day as I was paying for some purchases at a health food store I noticed a box of instant ginseng packets near the cash register, with a price tag of twenty-five cents per packet. That's a lot of money for one little envelope of powdered root, but I was in a daring mood and parted with a quarter to satisfy my curiosity about this famous plant, which I knew only by reputation.

When I got home I emptied the foil envelope and poured its contents into a mug. My twenty-five cents worth of ginseng was a teaspoon of gold-colored granules, of very regular size and shape. I filled the cup with hot water, noticed that the granules dissolved instantly, and took a sip.

Wow! The taste was superb. Ginseng tea snaps

you to attention in a subtle way, clearing the sinuses with a faint licorice-like aroma, and leaving you with the relaxed feeling of satisfaction which only a truly great hot beverage can produce.

Now, at least once a day, I tear open a ginseng tea packet and enjoy thoroughly its pungent, natural taste. And, rather strangely, the more ginseng I drink, the more I hanker to own one of those man-shaped roots.

Many other people have become ginseng fanciers, too. There has always been a small market for the root in U. S. health food stores, but now the trend is really up. Almost every store carries a selection of ginseng products in various forms and packages. The instant granules are the most popular, but ginseng liquid is also widely used. True, the cost is high, but the value is there even if you judge ginseng only on its flavor. After all, you have to pay fifteen cents or more these days for a bad cup of coffee in a restaurant, so why not sip the drink of Oriental kings for twenty-five cents in the privacy of your own home?

Much of the ginseng sold here in packaged form comes from Korea, which is somewhat of a turn-about. The U. S. used to be a prime supplier of wild ginseng root to the Orient, China in particular. Starting well before the Civil War, mountain folk combed the Appalachian hills and the woods of many eastern states, probing the deep hardwood shade for the mature roots of "seng," as they called it. The collectors themselves might earn several dollars a day, which was a good wage in this country a century ago. Most of the money in the ginseng trade, though, was probably earned by the Chinese buyers who set up shop in New York, Philadelphia, Cincinnati and other towns. Although those dealers bought a pound for five dollars or more, the warlords back in Chungking and Hangshow undoubtedly paid a much stiffer price for what they considered the medicine *par excellence,* the treatment of last resort for use when all other drugs had failed.

Today, the only wild seng left is growing, I am told, in snake-infested corners of the woods which are frequented by only a handful of determined wild-plant collectors.

What about growing some ginseng in your own garden, having fun in the process, and making a few dollars on the side? That idea is not at all new. In fact, well before the supplies of wild seng began to peter out, hobbyists and farmers were diligently trying to find a way to grow this much-desired plant commercially.

There are places in the United States where you can buy 1,000 ginseng seeds at prices ranging from $8.50 to $55, depending on whose advertisement you answer. And at least one company sells 100 "Strong Planting Roots (1-year seedlings)" for $16.75.

Dealers in the roots and seed will send out pamphlets telling briefly how to establish a ginseng garden. But in my opinion, the best source of information is the paperback book *Ginseng and Other Medicinal Plants* by A. R. Harding. It was originally published in 1908 and, the copyright having expired, is being issued in reprint form by Emporium Publications, P.O. Box 207, Boston, Massachusetts 02129. The price is four dollars, and you may be able to find it for sale in a large bookstore specializing in paperbacks.

Harding's ginseng book is worth owning if your interest is such that you contemplate trying to grow ginseng. I can't think of any question about its cultivation that isn't dealt with by Harding, and many aspects of ginseng culture are discussed several times by different farmers and article-writers who are quoted.

Although Harding's book doesn't try to hide the difficulties of ginseng growing, it says that the plant is of much interest to the average gardener. If you want to give it a try on a small scale yourself, start with the biggest, freshest roots you can get—not seeds. And if you do have hopes of recouping your investment or making some money, plan on harvesting seeds after a few years, which you may be able to sell to interested neighbors.

If you need a more solid reason to become interested in ginseng, consider the possibility that researchers may soon prove this honored and treasured plant really does have medicinal value.

Russian Scientists Explore New Ideas

The Russians have laboratories researching everything from astrological methods of sex selection of children to photography that reveals the psychic energy of people under different circumstances. And for years they have been working to find the true medicinal value of plants.

For example, the Russians were the first to pinpoint scientifically the specific health-giving values of garlic. And at least one herb book in my library indicates that Russian scientists have found that radiations given off by garlic are similar to those of ginseng.

More recently, the Russians have been trying to promote a plant of their own, *eleutherococcus senticosus,* which they claim has characteristics very much like ginseng. I. I. Brekhman, M.D., author of a book on *eleutherococcus,* recently made these rather interesting comments about it:

"By its pharmacological properties, *eleutherococcus* is in many features similar to ginseng. It is a stimulant, increasing the general tone of the organ-

61

ism, normalizing the arterial pressure and reducing an elevated blood sugar level. Owing to its capacity to strengthen the protective forces of the organism and to increase resistance against various adverse effects, *eleutherococcus* may be regarded as representative of those rare substances which possess an adaptogenic action, and contribute to the realization of its adaptive, 'protective' reaction of the organism." In other words, they say the *eleutherococcus* helps people resist the bad effects of stress more effectively.

What is the real truth about ginseng and this related Russian "super herb?" Are they beneficial plants, or is ginseng just a remarkably good-tasting root that has gotten along on a false reputation for several thousand years? I can't give you a positive answer, but I think you will enjoy exploring the world of plant therapeutics more thoroughly, and I suggest that ginseng is worth knowing, and perhaps growing.

BOOKS ON HEALING WITH HERBS

Earth Medicine—Earth Foods, Weiner, Michael A., The Macmillan Company, New York, 1972.

Encyclopedia of Medicinal Herbs, Kadans, Joseph M., Arco Publishers, New York, 1972.

Herbs Growing for Health, Law, Donald, ARC Books, 1969.

Herbcraft, Schafer, Violet, Yerba Buena Press, San Francisco, 1971.

The Herb Book: How to Use, Grow and Buy Nature's Miracle Plants. Edited by William H. Hylton, Rodale Press, 1974.

Using Plants for Healing, Coon, Nelson, Hearthside Press, Inc., 1963.

LET'S TAKE A NEW LOOK AT MEAT 5

Which is more healthful—a meat diet or a vegetarian diet? Vegetarians point to many reasons to back up their belief that non-meat foods are superior. Man is not a carnivore, they say. We were intended by nature to eat seeds and nuts, fruits and other parts of plants. Vegetarians cite the plant-eating gorilla as evidence that this kind of diet can produce a great physical strength. (Recently it has been found that gorillas eat small animals as well as plants.)

But most nutritionists are firm in saying that a diet should include meat. There is little doubt that it provides the best kind of protein, in ample amounts.

Although many leaders in the health movement have tended toward vegetarianism, the Rodale position has always been that meat adds both nutritional quality and flavor to the diet. My father, J. I. Rodale, thought that meat gave a person extra vigor. He tried in his youth to follow a vegetarian diet and found it unsatisfying. He was forced to eat more bread and sweet foods to make up for the calories he lost by not eating meat, and gradually began to feel sluggish and out of sorts. He switched back to meat and again enjoyed good health. That experience strongly influenced his views, and made him a confirmed meat-eater for the rest of his life.

63

There are other reasons why J. I. Rodale recommended meat so strongly. Twenty years ago meat was a much better product than it is today. Many animals were raised on family farms where they were given natural food. Meat animals were seldom given the chemical stimulants, hormones, antibiotics, and even arsenicals which are so commonly used today in animal and poultry feeds. They were not packed into feedlots, or herded into solitary-confinement cages. They were free to wander in fields and eat the grass.

Even then, vegetables and fruits were often grown in chemically fertilized soil and sprayed with insecticides. Vegetarians, J. I. Rodale thought, were hurting themselves by eating this food that had been sprayed, or treated with additives.

As we all know, the shoe is now on the other foot. Or perhaps it's better to say that the chemicalized shoes are on both feet. Most of the meat that you get in stores today is not nearly the quality it was 20 or even 10 years ago. High energy rations, supplemented with hormones and other boosters, transform much of the beef and chicken into products laden with water and lacking in taste. And worse is the worry that some of the chemicals used for fattening animals are still in the meat you eat.

Of course, fruits and vegetables are still likely to contain chemical residues unless they are organically grown, but you can no longer say that meat automatically enjoys an advantage when it comes to purity.

Of direct concern to most people is the dollars-and-cents cost of meat in today's supermarkets. Chicken continues to be pretty much of a bargain (not considering the chemicals and the lack of flavor). Putting steak, roasts, and even hamburger on the table can be a severe drain on the family budget.

But protein is essential to health and is an important element in well-balanced and abundant nutrition.

No single food of plant origin can match the protein quality and quantity of food that comes from animals.

Perhaps the protein goodness of beef and other meat has been oversold. Although eating meat is insurance against protein deficiency, *you don't have to eat a great deal of meat to get all the protein you need.* All that you have to do is eat the right combination of other foods.

We Should All Eat More Vegetables

I believe we should all be eating more fresh vegetables. They can make us healthier, just as our mothers told us when we were children. It is a matter of record that vegetable consumption in the United States has been on a steady downward course for generations.

During the period 1935 to 1939, American diets included an average of thirty pounds of vegetables a year. In 1965, the most current year for which we can find statistics, people ate only twenty-four pounds of vegetables a year. That figure doesn't include potatoes, incidentally.

Even so, twenty-four pounds of vegetables a year is a small amount for the average person to eat, when you consider that America's John Doe in 1965 ate 258 pounds of meat, fish, poultry, eggs and legumes, 237 pounds of dairy products, 51 pounds of fats, 168 pounds of fruit, 147 pounds of cereal and 112 pounds of sweets. Not only is there a small amount of vegetables bought and cooked, but I'm sure that many vegetables that reach the plate are prepared so poorly that they aren't consumed.

Another factor downgrading the beneficial effect of vegetables on the American diet is that they are served in strange, additive-laden ways dreamed up

by makers of convenience foods. For example, a
Boise, Idaho company tested a packaged food called
Garden Fries, which they label as "Carrots for people
who like French fries." The carrots are ground up
then blended with a modified food starch, flour,
spices and artificial butter flavor before being deep-
fried and frozen. What are good, old American
vegetables coming to?

You don't *have* to go the packaged vegetable
route. In fact, you shouldn't if you want the maximum health benefit from eating produce. The important thing is to start looking at vegetables as more
than just a decoration for the meat on your plate.
They truly are low in fat, high in protein, vitamins,
minerals and other valuable nutrients, especially
when served either raw or partially cooked. Vitamin
C, for which vegetables are highly valued, is sensitive
to heat and is depleted seriously during cooking at
high temperatures. Steaming vegetables is probably
the best way to cook them, if you must cook them at
all, since only a tiny amount of water is necessary for
steaming. If you do cook vegetables in water, be sure
to save the cooking water for use in soups or stews,
because it contains valuable nutrients.

If you have a sharp eye for research reports, it's
not hard to spot other indications that there's something in vegetables which the big meat-eaters may be
missing. For example, the *Los Angeles Times* of November 9, 1972 carried this story under the intriguing
headline: "Vegetables in Diet May Cut Cancer Risk."

"A group of scientists has found that people who
eat uncooked vegetables appear to have less stomach
cancer than the general population.

"Lettuce, tomatoes, carrots, coleslaw and red
cabbage in particular were found to be associated
with low risk of gastric cancer.

"The risk declined as the amount of these raw

vegetables eaten increased.

"Dr. Saxon Graham of the State University of New York at Buffalo, in an interview, said the findings came as a surprise and he was at a loss to explain the apparent protective effect of raw vegetables."

Although medical scientists don't study vegetables as diligently as they look for miracle drugs, nevertheless findings about the health-giving value of vegetables pop into the literature from time to time. About 10 years ago, scientists found that naval recruits from the mountainous regions of North and South Carolina had better teeth than young men from other parts of the country joining that service. After checking on the kind of food the recruits had been eating, the doctors concluded that the young men's high intake of dark-green leafy vegetables was an important factor in their superior dental health.

Some scientists actually have a fixation on the value of one specific vegetable. Ancel Keys, a big name in nutrition, believes that beans of all types are essential to heart health. In fact, he has written a book, *The Benevolent Bean,* in which he backs up that contention and provides numerous recipes aimed at encouraging his readers to eat more beans.

Keys points to the superior heart health of those Italians who eat a lot of beans—which incidentally were brought to Italy many years ago by explorers returning from America. One of the chief values of beans is the high content of unrefined carbohydrates, which supply energy without upsetting the body's balance of blood fats, as the refined carbohydrate sugar is thought to do by some doctors.

Corn is another amazing food. It offers great quantities of good quality protein, vitamins, minerals, roughage, and the unrefined carbohydrates that we need to be healthy. Corn is also cheap. Yet most people eat only token quantities of sweet corn, which is just one type of this valuable, native-American vegetable.

We can save plenty of money, reduce the amount of fat in our diets, and benefit in other ways by eating more corn. Our ancestors used meal from field corn as a staple part of their diet. They ate it every day in the form of corn bread, mush, fried mush, spoon bread and biscuits. Cornmeal kept them going, winter and summer.

Why don't we eat more corn today? Probably because it's too cheap and has no status value. Even bought at retail, in small packages, good cornmeal costs about ten cents a pound. One pound can supply the average family with pancakes for breakfast, biscuits for lunch and polenta for supper.

Bulk—A Unique Prize, A Vital Element

Natural, unprocessed vegetable foods contain a unique prize, a vital element notably lacking in the diets of most Americans—bulk; some call it "roughage" or crude fiber. No matter how you refer to it, fiber is that part of food that our bodies cannot absorb to use as fuel. Passing through the intestinal tract unscathed, it yields no vitamins, protein or calories. Yet, the natural fiber in whole, unprocessed foods may be instrumental in keeping cholesterol levels low and preventing the onset of heart disease. That's the opinion of Dr. Hugh Trowell, who spent years in Uganda studying the amazing health of rural Africans.

"Almost all Africans south of the Sahara eat natural carbohydrates or lightly processed cereals" like millet, Dr. Trowell reported recently in *The American Journal of Clinical Nutrition*. Seeds, groundnuts, and fibrous vegetables such as sweet potatoes are also featured heavily in the African diet. All of these items are good sources of fiber.

Our food, on the other hand, is largely refined carbohydrate which contains little crude fiber. Ever since the introduction in the last century of roller mills to process grain, Western man hasn't been getting much cereal fiber in his diet at all. While every 100 grams of whole wheat bread contains two grams of fiber, commercial white bread contains none at all, Dr. Trowell reports.

"Our Western ancestors ate 600 grams of whole-meal bread daily . . ." he says. "Africans, who were my patients for 30 years, still eat approximately two-thirds of their calories in unprocessed foods or lightly-milled maize. They get very little coronary heart disease or diverticular (lower bowel) disease."

To prove his point, Dr. Trowell cites an experiment in which a daily ration of chick peas supplying 16 grams of fiber successfully lowered the cholesterol counts of Indians eating a *high fat diet.* And in another study with Dutch volunteers, 140 grams of high-in-fiber rolled oats reduced cholesterol levels significantly in just three weeks.

Other researchers are convinced that adequate dietary fiber can also prevent such ailments as cancer of the colon, appendicitis, ulcerative colitis and diverticular disease.

The many vitamins stored in vegetables add to the reasonableness of cultivating a diet that is not dependent on meat. But don't take it for granted that all vegetables available provide the same fantastic vitamin quality of vegetables grown in your own garden. Some people have to live entirely on store-bought produce that has been carted half way across the country and piled in warehouses for as long as two or three weeks. Even worse off are the people who live entirely on restaurant food. The art of cooking vegetables lightly, to preserve their nutritional values, seems to be unknown today even in the finest and most expensive restaurants.

Not only can you assure freshness by growing your own vegetables, but now you can select types of plants that offer much greater nutritional values than the standardized, machine-harvested varieties grown on most commercial vegetable farms. The hard, poor-tasting, devitaminized tomatoes have become standard in most stores and the same sort of decline has afflicted other vegetables, too. Plant breeders have been selecting new types for qualities other than the ability to deliver vitamins to your table. Fortunately, the seed catalogs still offer the nutritious old-timers, plus even a few new types that are specially created for superior vitamin values in home-garden use. Hopefully, more such vegetables will be coming along in the future.

Avoid Meat Completely?

I am not advocating a *complete* vegetable-food diet. Such a diet presents serious nutritional problems. There are some people who won't even use eggs, cheese or milk. Largely for religious or philosophic reasons, these people eat only foods of plant origin. They are called vegans, and are frequently deficient in vitamin B_{12}, one vitamin that only animal products can supply in liberal quantities.

Seventh Day Adventists are required by their religion to follow a vegetarian diet, but they do eat eggs and dairy products. They have their own hospitals and a medical school, and they have been the subject of careful health surveys by researchers anxious to determine the physical effects of a meatless diet.

Male Seventh Day Adventists have 40 percent less coronary heart disease than the general population. Their overall health is significantly better than average. Female Seventh Day Adventists enjoy similar health benefits. Of course, non-smoking and avoidance of alcohol is also a part of their regimen, but vegetarianism must be an important factor in their good health.

Seventh Day Adventists do tend to have higher serum triglyceride levels than other people. That was reported by Richard T. Walden in the February, 1964, issue of the *American Journal of Medicine.* Serum triglycerides are usually elevated when people eat more refined carbohydrates, like sugar and possibly white flour.

My recommendation is to cut down drastically on steaks, chops, roasts, and chicken dinners. Americans are meat gluttons. Many people eat meat at every meal, a senseless overindulgence. Our national consumption of all meat products is way above the level that is necessary to supply an adequate diet. And because meat tends to be fatty and high in calories, a steady diet of beef and pork can put on extra pounds.

Eggs especially are great food. Their reputation as a cause of cholesterol problems is largely undeserved. So whatever you do, eat some eggs and natural cheese if you are inclined toward a complete no-meat diet.

Once you deliberately limit the amount of meat you eat, you gradually find yourself making a psychological adjustment. The important thing is to take that first step—to start eating some lunches and dinners that feature no beef or pork or chicken at all. Substitute whole, natural foods—not white bread and sweet desserts. Start that habit and you'll probably realize eventually that a juicy steak is not the be-all and end-all of good eating. I've made that adjustment, and look forward to meatless meals. I eat meat not so much by choice, but because it is put in front of me or because some restaurants can offer little else. I don't think that I will ever become a vegetarian, and I certainly won't be a vegan. But I'm eating a lot less meat, and enjoying my meals more.

Avoiding the Dangers of Vegetarianism

Eating more sugar to get the calories not supplied by meat is perhaps the greatest danger of vegetarianism—not protein deficiency. Therefore, if you start reducing your meat consumption, you must be extra careful to avoid junk foods. Be rigorous in cutting down on sugar and white flour as well as meat. Stay away from all desserts that are not fresh fruits, seeds, or whole grains. And don't be misled by the protein claims that are made for the highly-advertised commercial breakfast cereals. Very often this protein is actually less available to you than the manufacturers claim, because the heavy processing of those products makes their protein more difficult to assimilate.

Cutting out the bad foods entirely and replacing them with natural foods, like whole grains, natural cheese, eggs, salads, seeds and fruits, largely relieves you of the need to calculate your protein intake. If you eat only good food, using your natural common sense to define what good food is, there is hardly any likelihood that you will have to worry about getting sufficient protein while eating less meat.

However, many health-minded people want a more precise way of knowing the nutritional value of what they eat, including protein. For these people,

I recommend the paperback book, *Diet for a Small Planet* by Frances Moore Lappé, published by Ballantine Books. In the first half of her book Mrs. Lappé describes quite plainly and understandably how healthful protein is made from a combination of amino acids. She tells how you can know which foods have which amino acids, and how to combine foods of non-meat origin to be sure to get the proper protein balance. Mrs. Lappé's thrust is that we are a nation that squanders protein by eating too much meat, thereby causing harm to our environment and exposing ourselves to needless health risks.

An important rule to keep in mind about protein from plant sources is to eat at each meal food that comes from different parts of plants. In other words, try to combine leaves, seeds, stems and roots of different vegetable plants at one meal. Each part of the plant tends to have a different amino acid balance, so by eating all parts at one time you get protein that is close to being highest quality, and completely balanced.

Remember that it's necessary to eat balanced protein at each meal. In other words, you can't eat beans for lunch and rice for supper and expect to get the wonderful protein quality of a beans-and-rice meal. Your lunchtime beans will be digested and on their way through your gut by the time the supper time rice enters your stomach. So stress variety at each meal, eating different foods instead of filling up on one food.

Keep an open mind and give some of these meal plans a try. I'm sure you will find the benefits rewarding.

REVELATIONS FROM A LOCK OF HAIR 6

Next time you get a haircut, think of those clippings on the floor not as waste but as a record of your trace element nutrition—and possibly your current health status. Scientists, in increasing numbers, are looking at hair as a useful recording filament that can help solve important health problems.

The growing realization of the importance of trace elements is the reason for the new interest in hair. A person needs regular but small amounts of nutrients like zinc, copper, manganese and magnesium to stay healthy—and also he must be careful to avoid overexposure to harmful elements like lead. Studies have shown that those trace elements have significant effects not only on our susceptibility to disease, but also on our rate of growth, the way we feel, and even on our intelligence.

When A. S. Prasad began his now-classic investigation on the reasons for growth patterns of Egyptian dwarfs, in 1963, he had a number of diagnostic methods at his disposal. He studied the dwarfs' outward symptoms, their retarded growth and stunted sexual development. He studied their diet to see what critical nutrient might possibly be lacking. He studied their blood plasma in the laboratory to determine what elements were at a low level.

Those were all traditional diagnostic tools, used for years by trained epidemiologists.

But Prasad had still another scientific tool, a comparatively new one, that few had used before him and no one had used in precisely his manner. Prasad was able to detect the dwarfs' critical zinc deficiency *by analyzing their hair!*

Scientists now know that zinc levels in normal human hair can run from 125 to 200 parts per million. Prasad found that the hair zinc levels of the dwarfs averaged a meager 54 ppm. However, when the dwarfs were treated with oral zinc sulfate and placed on better diets, their hair zinc levels shot up into the normal range.

By probing the mysteries in a strand of hair, Prasad was opening up new chapters in scientific detective work. As zinc authority William Strain commented a few years later, "The application of hair analysis to the diagnosis of zinc deficiency in the Egyptian dwarfs was the first demonstration of the value of using hair analysis as a means of estimating human zinc stores."

How is human hair analyzed? The technique is known as Atomic Absorption Analysis. The researcher clips about a tablespoon of hair from the nape of the subject's neck. This sample is then washed repeatedly in detergent and distilled water, then ashed or "digested" with acids. The residue is analyzed to determine its content of a given mineral element—in this case, zinc.

But why hair? Like the concentric rings of growth on a proud old tree, every strand of growing hair carries with it an impression, an exact record of the body's health and nutrition back into the past. If you want to know your nutritional state last week, you must analyze the hair closest to the scalp. If you're curious about your body's health a month, or perhaps even a year ago, you analyze the extremities of the hair strands.

The idea of atomic absorption analysis of hair or blood is not new. It was first proposed in 1859 by G. R. Kirchhoff. Later, in 1882, it was described in Schellen's book, *Spectrum Analysis*. But the actual technique was not really perfected until 1955 when A. Walsh, an Australian physicist, developed the instruments and techniques necessary to do the job.

Amazing as it may seem now, the new tool was generally ignored by scientists in the United States while researchers in other nations forged ahead with it. That temporary disinterest once prompted Walsh to comment that the United States was, at least in one sense, an underdeveloped nation.

But within the last decade or so, hair analysis by the method I described has become quite common in this country. Ironically, much of the impetus for its use came as a response to environmental pollutants, rather than from any desire to study human nutrition.

Scientists have found that potentially dangerous trace pollutants such as lead, cadmium, mercury and arsenic are often concentrated in human hair. In fact, by analyzing the metal content of hair, we can now accurately determine the exposure of an individual or an entire community to various poisons in the atmosphere.

Dr. D. I. Hammer of the Ecological Research Board, Environmental Health Service, Durham, North Carolina, is one scientist who has been very active in this field. Human hair, he says, may prove to be "a practical dosimeter for many environmental pollutants."

In similar fashion, scientists around the world are analyzing the mercury content of human hair for clues to pollution sickness. In Japan, the mercury content of scalp hair has been determined in patients with Minamata disease, a consequence of industry's dumping mercury wastes into local waters. Another Japanese study has shown a strong link between hair's mercury content and the amount of mercury-contaminated fish a person has consumed. In Sweden, chest hair has been analyzed to gauge similar exposure in fishing communities. And researchers in America have found that people in industrial urban areas have higher hair levels of mercury than those in nonindustrial rural and suburban areas.

The fine art and science of hair analysis has been perfected to such a point that Canadian criminal researchers now boast that by testing a person's hair for 18 key trace metals, they can produce a hair profile as unique as a fingerprint.

Hair analysis can be a tool for dietary improvement too, as we've seen in the case of zinc. Because hair is composed largely of protein, it can easily be used to detect malnourishment. The hair shaft narrows in malnutrition just like the limbs of an underfed child, says Dr. R. G. Crounse of the Medical College of Georgia.

Using hair analysis, nutritionist Robert Bradfield of the University of California at Berkeley has developed an "early warning system" for detecting marasmus and kwashiorkor, two deadly protein deficiency diseases that afflict children in underdeveloped lands. Bradfield has found that under the microscope, hair roots and shafts show damage weeks before protein deficiency can be detected otherwise. Instead of waiting for the telltale symptoms—withered limbs, swollen bellies and deficient blood—a doctor using hair analysis can start treating these unfortunate children immediately. Pediatricians in New Guinea are already using Bradfield's technique to screen children for protein deficiency.

But dramatic as these findings are, perhaps no

nutritional element is more intimately bound up with the new science of hair analysis than zinc. That mineral gained its current prominence as a vital health factor largely through information gained by hair analysis. Without it, it is doubtful that we would realize, as we now do, that zinc can influence the way children grow, the way some diseases are resisted, and even how people feel. The method is painless, rapid, accurate and inexpensive, making it possible to do large-scale sampling for a variety of trace minerals.

Not only is hair testing a good way to diagnose zinc deficiency, but hair itself is also influenced by the amount of zinc in the body. Agricultural scientists have known for years that zinc-deficient feed causes animals to lose their hair and develop scaly skin. When zinc supplements are introduced into the feed of animals, their hair and skin health are restored. In his important book *Mineral Nutrition and the Balance of Life,* Professor Frank A. Gilbert notes that "Zinc deficient animals in tests had a greatly retarded growth rate, became emaciated, and lost hair." The same thing happens with birds, who show poor condition of their feathers when fed a zinc-deficient diet.

Although there haven't yet been any large-scale tests on the effects of extra zinc nutrition on the hair health of people, numerous reports of hair improvement in animals have led some scientists to conduct informal experiments on themselves—with very interesting results. P. N. Demertzis of the Research Laboratory of Physiopathology of Animal Reproduction in Athens, Greece, wrote of his personal experiences in a letter to the journal, *The Lancet,* published in the December 9, 1972, issue.

"Working recently with zinc," he said, "I was impressed with the effect of zinc supplements on apparently healthy animals. So I decided to take zinc myself. The result was surprising. Firstly, the long hairs of the eyebrows (a sign of the aged) disappeared and new, short, and thin adolescent-like eyebrows took their place. The hair became more healthy and shining, its color darker, and every trace of dandruff disappeared. In the comb in the morning there was not a single hair any more. Finally the greasy skin (full of acne at the time of my adolescence) became dry and better than I had ever had it.

"After my experience, the same effect was noted in three other people I know, who took zinc."

Why does improved zinc nutrition help to improve the quality of hair? That's still partly a mystery, and more research is needed. However, there are signs that zinc—a remarkably friendly and healing element—is one of those things, like vitamin C and vitamin E, where the amount necessary to prevent outright deficiency is short of the amount sufficient to achieve the maximum beneficial effect.

For a long time scientists were saying that there's no such thing as zinc deficiency in people, that the 15 milligrams we supposedly need each day are easily obtainable from food. But now we are finding that those 15 milligrams *aren't* so readily obtained from foods grown with heavy applications of chemical fertilizers, which tend to *reduce* zinc content in plants.

The boom in zinc interest among nutritional scientists is turning up increasing evidence that those people who have more than average amounts of zinc in their systems enjoy positive benefits—not limited to a better head of hair. One of the most exciting such reports comes from Adon A. Gordus, Ph.D., professor of chemistry at the University of Michigan. Right now, he is in the middle of perhaps the largest hair-testing research project of all time. In order to find out how much industrialization and modern living has changed human trace element nutrition and exposure over the past few generations, he is checking 1400 samples of human hair collected from people who died many years ago. Each sample is tested for 38 different elements. For comparison, Professor Gordus has collected and is analyzing the hair of students at two service academies, the University of Michigan and other schools.

A remarkable pattern soon emerged from the test results of the modern samples: high zinc content in the hair and better marks in school go together! "It appears that those students with the highest grade-point average frequently tend to have higher than normal zinc and copper content in their hair, but lower than normal iodine content," Professor Gordus reported at the recent national meeting of the American Chemical Society.

"Hair may also prove to be an indicator of the rate of metabolic adjustment to a new environment," he observed. "For example, it might show how fast a person can get rid of a dangerous chemical once that chemical has been removed from his intake." Gordus also said the researchers hope eventually to compare the hair content of healthy individuals with that of people with certain diseases, particularly those of a neurological nature. He noted that the diagnostic role hair might play is enhanced by its unique concentrating ability. Mercury content in hair, for example, is about 200 to 300 times that of human blood.

Pointing out that food is the major source of trace elements, Professor Gordus said the hair of male Eskimos was compared with that of dark-haired servicemen of similar age. "The gross difference in diet showed up quite clearly in the tests," the Michigan professor reported. The Eskimos' hair contained considerably more arsenic, magnesium, iodine, and other elements associated with the extensive consumption of salt-water fish and mammals. Conversely, the servicemen's hair contained more calcium, probably from drinking more milk, and chromium. Gordus speculated that the higher chromium content might be due to the processing of foods in stainless steel vessels. While not necessarily dangerous, ingredients in certain foods cause the release of some chromium from stainless steel.

Hair snipped from male and female college students of similar age also differs, tests show. Gordus said that women's hair seems to have more calcium, iodine and aluminum, while male hair has decidedly more manganese.

Preliminary analyses of some of the 1,400 historic hair samples already collected indicate a higher arsenic content, Gordus noted. "The arsenic in the older hair might not have been ingested," he said. "Most of the samples are from rural, largely unindustrialized areas, and the insecticides used in the past contained a lot of arsenic." He noted that most cases of abnormally high concentrations of elements encountered in modern hair could be traced to external overexposure, such as selenium from a scalp medication or bromine and copper from treated swimming pools.

Can taking zinc make you smarter? Professor Gordus isn't sure. "It's entirely possible that those of higher intelligence simply excrete more zinc," he says, pointing out that an extensive study is needed to find out for certain what is happening. His connection between large units of zinc in the hair and improved intelligence is not an isolated finding. Several experiments have shown that giving animals more zinc in their diet actually makes them smarter!

The most interesting work in this area has been done by Donald Oberleas, Ph.D. and his colleagues at the medical school of Wayne State University in

Detroit. In a study published in the *Psychopharmacology Bulletin,* July, 1971 they reported that zinc-supplemented rats "exhibited a superior rate of learning." They were able to learn their way through a maze more quickly than rats not given a zinc-supplemented diet. Dr. Oberleas was encouraged to conduct his experiment by previous zinc nutrition studies which had shown that "in both animals and men, deficient subjects appeared more listless and lethargic." It certainly is reasonable to assume that there is a close connection between listlessness and inability to learn.

Carrying his work further, Dr. Oberleas raised female rats on a diet mildly deficient in zinc. Not only did they have smaller litters and poorer milk production than normal rats, but their offspring suffered significant and permanent behavioral changes. They couldn't cope with a maze or other intelligence tests as well as normal rats.

Another experiment, showing the effect of zinc supplementation on human intelligence, was described by Dr. Oberleas in a letter to *Chemical and Engineering News,* July 10, 1972:

"There is one other account (on zinc) in humans which was reported by Dr. H. A. Ronaghy in a symposium in Cleveland in October of last year. That particular study was done with 19-20 year old human zinc-deficient subjects in Iran. These subjects were illiterate at the beginning of the study, but there was a marked differential in scholastic performance after one year in the zinc-supplemented subjects."

Think for a moment of what is happening. Our diet is becoming more zinc deficient year by year, largely because of the overuse of synthetic fertilizers and changing eating habits. And now we know that zinc deficiency is closely allied with loss of intelligence—and may even be irreversible! The Roman

Empire fell, some experts say, because the aristocracy drank wine from leaden jars, causing lead poisoning on a massive scale. In a similar way, we could eventually lose our position of world leadership because we don't get enough zinc in our food to stay as smart as people who eat naturally fertilized food.

Run your fingers through your hair as you ponder that thought. Your hair, in fact, may be the answer—our salvation—because in everyone's hair is a record of how much zinc they have been getting over a period of time. Of course, all parts of our bodies contain zinc in varying degrees. It circulates in our blood, accumulates in our bones, and is excreted in our wastes.

Hair has much to recommend it as a test-base for any mineral element in the body. It is easy to collect, for one thing. With blood tests, a nurse has to use a needle to collect a sample, which means not only a trip to a clinic but a moment of unpleasantness. Hair can be clipped easily by anyone. Besides being easy to obtain, hair is easy to store and ship in hot, humid climates where blood and other living tissues quickly deteriorate.

Another important advantage in using hair for trace element testing is that it *reflects the trace element status over a reasonable period of time.* The composition of blood changes from hour to hour, depending on what you have eaten recently, or on other types of stress. Hair, on the other hand, grows a little each day, and each day's growth reflects the nutritional status of your body on that particular day.

William Strain, Ph.D., a leader in the use of hair analysis in zinc research, found that one burn victim had 300 parts per million of zinc in the long hair, but only 47 parts per million in the short hair at the nape of the neck.

Bone would be a good part of the body to test

for trace elements because bone is where we store many of these minerals. The elements collected there provide a permanent lifetime record of mineral nutrition. But bone has two serious disadvantages over hair for testing. First, samples are very difficult to collect from living people. And second, a test of bone would reflect mineral nutrition over too long a time. A hair test tells how much of an element you have been getting in the past few weeks or months, which could be far more important.

Of course, hair testing is a fairly new science. It has been done on such a small scale that there is still a certain amount of doubt about the levels of trace elements in hair that can be considered normal. There is also a lack of information about the effect of hair coloring, pollution, occupational exposure and other factors on hair analysis. But those questions remain puzzling mainly because the number of hair tests that have been made is very small. As the technique comes into wider use, the amount of data on what is normal will increase and the tests can be interpreted with more certainty.

Even the small amount of hair testing that has been done up to now has produced some quite interesting results. For example, Dr. Strain tested the hair of ten medical students from Stockholm, Sweden, picked at random, and compared them with hair tests made on ten samples collected from ten medical students living in Rochester, New York. He found that the Swedish students had definitely higher amounts of zinc in their hair. Swedes enjoy better health than Americans, a fact usually attributed to social factors. Dr. Strain has another idea. "The better health of Swedish citizens may be due to an increased dietary intake of zinc through high consumption of ocean fish and potatoes," he says.

A test made on my own hair recently showed

that I am well-endowed with zinc. My hair contained 210 parts per million, which is over the range that Dr. Strain has been using as normal—125 to 150 parts per million for men and 125 to 160 parts per million for women.

Why is my zinc level good? There are probably several reasons. First, I don't drink alcohol, with very rare exceptions. Alcohol literally flushes zinc out of the system. Second, I eat foods grown without the synthetic fertilizers that are causing most commercially available foods to be lower in zinc content. Third, I take plenty of bone meal, which contains some zinc—not enough to have it considered a zinc supplement for general use, but enough to help raise your zinc level somewhat. Fourth, I eat very little of the empty calorie foods—like sugar and refined flour —and instead concentrate on eating foods that tend to be good sources of trace elements. Fifth, I include some meat, fish and eggs, some of the best sources of zinc, in my diet.

Still, if and when natural zinc supplements are made available, I'm going to take them. On the basis of more data now available, Dr. Strain is raising his normal hair zinc levels to 125 to 200 parts per million for men, and 125 to 300 parts per million for females. That would put my reading of 210 parts per million just a trifle over normal. And as I've been pointing out, there's plenty of indication that zinc is associated with positive health advantages.

Essentially, the idea of hair analysis is both logical and right. Your hair is an extension of you. It grows from within your body, and its composition reflects the environment that you create for yourself by what you eat and how you live. Testing hair for content of trace elements is, in my opinion, going to be a very popular and useful tool for building a personalized health program. People who are interested in their health need a way to check on whether their diet and other health practices are truly helping them. Science has created many new tests to detect disease, but hardly any tests to help people find a way to improve their health. Hair analysis for trace elements may soon become that kind of widely useful health test.

ZINC—THE MIRACLE MINERAL OF TOMORROW 7

It's time to start thinking about a little-known trace element that can have an important effect on your health.

Each vitamin, mineral, trace element, enzyme, amino acid or other nutrient that's known to be necessary in the diet of healthy people has a story that can be told. Some, like vitamin C and vitamin E, have been written about many times. Others are still waiting to be discovered fully by a public anxious to know everything possible about what's important to health.

Zinc is one of those elements that's been largely ignored. There have been few articles about it in popular magazines and newspapers, and until recently even the nutrition scientists didn't pay much attention to it. Probably 999 out of 1,000 people don't even know that zinc is an essential element in the human diet.

There are two reasons why zinc has not attracted much attention. One reason is the belief that we need only a small amount each day—about 15 milligrams. The other is that it has been assumed, until quite recently, that no matter what foods you eat you're going to get all the zinc you need. That second assumption has now been proven wrong. In fact, there's

89

a strong possibility that millions of people are experiencing a wide variety of bothersome symptoms as a result of moderate to severe zinc deficiency.

Agricultural scientists have known for years that zinc deficiency is a problem on farm lands. As early as 1927, zinc fertilizers had proven beneficial on Florida vegetable crops, and since World War II the zinc shortage on soils has become much worse, showing up as widespread deficiencies.

Today, citrus crops of all kinds need zinc fertilizer to grow at their best, no matter where they are grown, as do grains, vegetables and fruits in thirty two states. Frank G. Vets, Jr., of the Agricultural Research Service of the U. S. Department of Agriculture wrote in the book *Zinc Metabolism* (Charles C. Thomas Company, 1966), that "In some western states, zinc deficiency is now regarded as serious, second only to nitrogen deficiency among soil fertility problems." And he notes that zinc deficiency is not only an American problem—it's worldwide, "steadily increasing in intensity and scope." He cites parts of Australia, New Zealand, South Africa, Western Europe and south-central Asia as among the "principal areas" of zinc deficiency in the soil.

Contrary to what the Food and Drug Administration implies in its new dietary food regulations, mineral deficiency in the soil does show up as mineral deficiency in plants, and can affect the health of people who eat those mineral-deficient foods. This is especially true of trace elements like zinc, and in fact the significant and continual decrease in the trace element levels of grain has been a problem of great concern to enlightened farmers, especially those who feed the crops they raise to their own animals.

The article "Trace Mineral Levels in Grains Dropping" in the December, 1969, issue of *National Hog Farmer* tells the story pretty well. It reports that hogs are getting stress syndrome—"they may shake and even go into convulsions and die"—as a result of lowering levels of some trace minerals in their feed. Iron and copper are principal concerns, but the article notes that the average level of zinc in corn dropped from 22.01 parts per million in 1966-67 to 19.90 parts in 1968—roughly one season. Large variations in zinc content from one sample of oats to another were found. (Oats are thought to be quite a good source of zinc.) Some samples of oats contained seventy parts per million of zinc while others were as low as 3.2 parts per million. That kind of variation is caused by difference in soil levels of zinc.

Why Zinc Levels in Plants and Foods Have Been Dropping

Very recently, the zinc deficiency problem in foods has been brought into close focus by two agricultural researchers at West Virginia University in Morgantown, Drs. Robert F. Keefer and Rabindar N. Singh. They found that low zinc levels appear in sweet corn when the soil in which the plants are grown is heavily treated with artificial fertilizers, particularly phosphorus and nitrogen. Their finding is exciting, and could provide the best clue to why zinc levels in various plants and foods have been dropping. The heavy applications of yield-boosting chemical fertilizers that farmers are applying, say the two researchers, put great strains on the soil's slender reserves of zinc and end up causing zinc-deficient food.

Of course, they point out that their research was done with just one plant—sweet corn—and "such deficiencies can easily be corrected with other foods." That's the standard view that pops up continually when a soil-related mineral deficiency is discovered, and undoubtedly does have a certain amount of merit. But many other crops, not just sweet corn, are experiencing the zinc pinch. As more of these studies are made, the same pattern of zinc deficiency caused by high use of artificial fertilizers is likely to show up in other food plants.

Even more convincing is the accumulating evidence that zinc deficiency has already caused health problems in American people, especially children. Dr. M. C. Michael Hambidge, a pediatrician at the University of Colorado Medical Center, found last year that a group of school children who had poor appetites, slow growth-rates and poor sense of taste and smell were actually suffering from severe zinc deficiency. They were not from poor families, and weren't thought to be malnourished or even unhealthy in the usual sense. Yet tests made from samples of their hair showed them to be zinc-deficient.

About eight percent of the children in the Colorado study fell into the zinc-deficient category, but the problem is probably much wider than that. "Marginal zinc nutrition is no longer an esoteric consideration as far as young American children are concerned," says Dr. Harold H. Sandstead of the U.S. Department of Agriculture's Human Nutrition Laboratory at Grand Forks, North Dakota. And although Dr. Sanstead, like most experts on zinc nutrition, feels that children are exposed to the greatest risk, his work concerns the effect of zinc intake on all age groups.

"There is ample reason to suspect that zinc intakes of a number of individuals in this country may be marginal," Dr. Richard W. Luecke told food technologists at an international symposium last summer. Dr. Luecke, a biochemist, claims that "Zinc shortages can be found in all people, rich or poor." Perhaps some might even benefit by taking a zinc pill to supplement their diet, he said.

Some of the most fascinating, and in a way frightening, new information about zinc nutrition comes from two researchers at Lafayette Clinic, an affiliate of the Wayne State University School of Medicine in Detroit. Dr. Donald F. Caldwell, a psychologist, and Dr. Donald Oberleas, a biochemist, have found that people who rely primarily on vegetable foods for their protein may not actually be absorbing all the protein they need, because of a lack of sufficient zinc in their systems. There is more zinc in meat and some fish than there is in plant origin foods. The body needs zinc to make use of protein (either plant protein or animal protein), and the seed foods which are often used as protein sources by vegetarians contain phytate (a chelator) which locks up zinc and makes it unavailable to the body.

The variety of foods that vegetarians eat in this country is probably great enough to prevent severe zinc deficiencies, but it is something to think about.

High Percentage of Americans Are Zinc-Deficient

Dr. Caldwell and Dr. Oberleas are not optimistic. As many as eighty percent of Americans are experiencing zinc deficiency in some way, they estimate. While it's impossible now to say how much zinc is enough, the two doctors point out that your body throws off zinc when you have a cold, or when you sweat profusely.

Food processing also cuts our chances of getting adequate zinc. Canning is detrimental to zinc levels of some foods, Henry A. Schroeder, M.D., has reported. According to his figures, spinach loses 40.1 percent of its zinc when canned. Beans lose 60 percent and tomatoes lose 83.3 percent. Refining of flour to make bread also reduces zinc. White bread has 77.4 percent less zinc than whole wheat bread.

What can lack of zinc do to your health and body processes? My introduction to this facet of the zinc question came one day about eight or nine years ago when I dropped into the University of Rochester laboratory of William H. Strain, Ph.D., one of the world's foremost zinc researchers. I was in Rochester on vacation, heard about Dr. Strain's work from a friend, and called to ask if I could pay him a visit.

"I'm busy with my rats," he said over the phone, "but you can come down here (he was in the basement) and talk to me while I inject them." So while he injected the veins of rats' tails with zinc solutions, I asked him questions about his work.

Bill Strain and his former student, Air Force Surgeon Walter Pories, were at that time concerned mainly with the ability of zinc supplements to speed the healing of wounds. For their tests they used the easily standardized operation on pilonidal sinuses, chronically inflamed pits at the base of the spine. They found that subjects given zinc sulfate therapy were almost completely healed after forty-six days, while others not medicated still had open wounds until eighty days on the average. "Healing is definitely promoted, perhaps to the optimum rate," they said in an article reporting their results.

Strain and Pories also found that zinc therapy was effective in speeding the healing of burns, helping people who suffered from leg pain as a result of intermittent claudication and possibly could play an important role in the prevention of atherosclerosis.

Bill Strain and Dr. Pories are now at Case Western Reserve University Medical School in Cleveland and are still working with zinc. They are studying imbalances of zinc and other elements associated with degenerative diseases. The search is for the mineral pattern that means good health and for mineral therapies that correct mineral deficiencies.

Other researchers are also actively looking for applications for zinc supplementation. Taste loss, a symptom of zinc deficiency, is getting more attention. Dr. Robert I. Henkin, of the National Heart and Lung Institute, said last year that doctors should consider taste loss more as a nutritional problem and resist classifying it as a psychiatric disorder. Dr. Henkin had 103 patients with the affliction, and gave them zinc supplements four times a day in doses of 25, 50 or 100 milligrams. "About two-thirds were normal following treatment and all had some improvement," he reported. Those who got the most zinc recovered most rapidly.

Zinc's Effect on the Body

It's important to realize that work on zinc nutrition is still in its early stages, and that much of it has been with animals, not people. Nevertheless, I will give you a list of some of the effects that scientists have reported as associated with zinc levels:

1. —Lethargy, apathy, an unwillingness to learn and a general "blah" attitude are associated with zinc deficiency, it was noted by the Wayne State psychologist, Dr. Donald F. Caldwell.

2. —Bone formation is helped by zinc supplementation, report Dr. N. R. Calhoun and associates at the V. A. Hospital, Washington, D.C.

3. —Zinc is vital for the digestion of proteins, helps your body use up lactic acid developed during exercise, and also helps undo the effects of alcohol, claims Dr. Jean Mayer, Harvard nutritionist, in one of his syndicated newspaper columns.

4. —Low levels of zinc have been associated with atherosclerosis in several studies. Analysis of the hair is used by Drs. Strain and Pories to reveal this effect.

—Therapy with zinc supplements was found to give dramatic benefit to some patients with severe atherosclerotic disease by J. H. Menzel, M.D., and his associates at the University of Missouri Medical Center in Columbia.

5. —Gum healing after tooth extraction was speeded by a combination of vitamins and zinc supplementation. That finding was reported by James F. Smith, D.D.S., and James Bell, M.D., of the University of Tennessee's Institute of Pathology.

Those are sound reasons for making sure we get enough zinc.

Basically, there are two ways for us to get zinc, through our food and from mined sources. Nutritionally, food is our most important source, but mined zinc is important too. Our zinc ore resources are quite limited. Right now, the U.S. is producing eighty-one percent of the zinc ore used for fertilizers, alloys, drugs, and other industrial purposes. The National Commission on Materials Policy recently reported that by the year 2000 we are going to have to be importing eighty-one percent of our zinc, because domestic supplies will have been so depleted and the demand will have increased.

High-Zinc Foods

What about high-zinc foods? By far the richest nutritional source of zinc is the oyster. That tasty little fellow, probably because he filters vast amounts of mineral-rich seawater through his system, contains about 100 times as much zinc as most other types of food. I don't advocate that you eat oysters, however, because you can pick up hepatitis and other viruses from them, especially when they are taken from polluted waters. Someone may be able to make a purified, natural zinc supplement from oysters, although that is likely to be expensive and available in limited quantity.

Herring is also reportedly zinc-rich. Herring meal is another possibility. We've estimated that one teaspoon of dried and powdered herring would provide an adequate amount of zinc for those people who wouldn't care to eat fish every day. Zinc gluconate, a naturally processed form of mined zinc, is also available as a supplement ingredient.

Supplements of zinc are important, and we believe that large numbers of people will ultimately be using them. But to me, the most important aspect of this whole story is the declining ability of our soils to deliver zinc to us in our foods.

And as far as I can determine, zinc is one of the few elements approaching the status of nutritional crisis as a result of soil deficiencies and related problems. True, other minerals are being depleted in plants because of declining fertility, but we can usually make up for those deficiencies quite easily by eating more mineral-rich foods. Zinc is a special case. The zinc-rich foods are odd things like oysters and herring, which few people would care to eat every day. So we desperately need to get as much zinc as possible in all our foods by encouraging the widespread use of farming methods that will produce high-nutrient crops.

We have faced a similar problem with iodine, which is deficient in some inland soils. This deficiency causes the inhabitants to be more susceptible to goiter unless they use iodized salt, or eat ocean fish regularly. The iodine problem is important too, but it doesn't have nearly the significance of zinc depletion of the soil.

Another indication of the importance of zinc to us is a statement made, by Donald Oberleas, Ph.D., and colleagues, to the Federation of American Societies for Experimental Biology last year. They pointed out that over thirty different enzymes are zinc-dependent, which is about three times as many as have been decribed as magnesium-dependent. "Those two elements (zinc and magnesium) are probably the most important non-hormonal metabolic regulators in the body and few metabolic pathways can be found which do not require one or both," Oberleas said. Lack of zinc therefore has an ominous potential for causing trouble.

The problems presented by a lack of iodine and those presented by a lack of zinc differ in another way, which is purely agricultural but still extremely important. Iodine is naturally low or missing in some soils. Zinc, as far as we know, originally was present in adequate amounts in almost all U.S. soils, but is being depleted or made unavailable to plants (and thereby to us) by agricultural practices.

Zinc Is Lost in the Shuffle of Synthetic Fertilizers

The overuse of cheap, synthetic nitrogen and phosphorus fertilizers is turning our farms into factories producing bulk food, not food of the highest quality. Plants are smothered by overloads of the major nutrients, causing roots to lose their ability to forage for all nutrients in a balanced way. Zinc is lost in the shuffle.

The Zinc Institute points that out. "Millions of acres of cropland and pasture are fertilized with zinc to insure maximum yields of crops and forage," it says in a booklet on animal nutrition. "Even so, the amounts of zinc are often too low for healthy growth of livestock and optimum feed efficiency."

There is evidence, however, that the techniques of organic farming provide a positive solution to the problem. Firman E. Bear, a famous soil scientist, has noted that zinc deficiency occurs mainly in soil low in organic matter. Organic matter helps improve plant nutrition in many ways. The humic acids it releases dissolve mineral particles that are locked up in the soil's reserves. Organic matter also buffers and stores available nutrients, allowing roots to absorb them in an orderly way, instead of being overwhelmed by sudden doses of soluble fertilizers.

Organic fertilizers, especially those made from garbage and sewage sludge, are good sources of zinc. Two technical reports from the January-March issue of the *Journal of Environmental Quality* show that such composts contain zinc, and when used as fertilizer are effective in increasing the zinc content of plants. Instead of wasting our garbage and sewage, we should make sure that it is returned to the land.

Another cause of zinc deficiency is the obsolescence of galvanized water pipes, buckets, tubs and other containers. Zinc is the main ingredient in galvanizing, and it's quite possible that small amounts of zinc migrated from galvanized coatings into our food stream, and served a useful nutritional purpose. It is a fact that acid foods, when stored in galvanized containers, can pick up enough zinc to cause stomach upsets. Fortunately, the effects of an overdose of zinc are mild, and not long-lasting. In fact, zinc expert Bill Strain says that 30 times the usual dosage is required before major toxic symptoms occur.

For thousands of years, people have used zinc compounds to heal skin problems. And though zinc has been widely used as a raw material in industry for centuries, it has presented few health problems.

Cancer researchers are impressed by the relative safety of zinc. Of all the substances that can stimulate the production of lymphocytes—infection-battling cells in our blood—zinc is the only one that occurs naturally in the human body. This was pointed out recently in *The Lancet* (June 9, 1973) by H. Kirchner of the National Cancer Institute in Bethesda, Maryland, who also reported that "adverse side-effects have not been observed after oral zinc medication."

Far more important than any question of toxicity are the many benefits which result from having sufficient zinc. The average American is probably limping along on less of this vital element than is necessary to achieve maximum health.

As I noted before, healing of wounds and injuries has been speeded dramatically by zinc supplementation. Anyone facing an operation, or waiting out the healing process of any injury, should try hard to build up zinc reserves.

Dr. Oberleas questions the almost automatic way in which many people eat cereal for breakfast, ignoring other foods which could supply equal or better nutrition and not contribute zinc-binding phytates to the diet. The accessibility of children to peanut butter in large quantities also leaves them open to zinc deficiency, he feels. And of great concern to him is the feeding of soy formulas, along with cereal, to infants who can't keep down regular milk. "That's difficult on their zinc balance," he says.

These may be hard concepts for some people to face. We natural food people love our whole grains, our natural peanut butter, and our unprocessed soybeans. My feeling is that there is no need to avoid these foods, as long as you are sure you're getting enough zinc from another source, such as a food supplement. Moderation is the key to a good diet, combined with an interest in finding out the basic facts of nutrition and a willingness to use supplements when conditions require them.

The evidence exists to show that trace elements can work health miracles. We already know that people who live in certain areas of the world, where the balance of mineral elements is favorable, live to very advanced ages and enjoy great vigor and freedom from disease. There is also evidence that people in some places have better teeth, or fewer heart attacks, or stronger bones—all because certain "minor" minerals are in the proper balance in their soil, food and water. What remains to be done—and it is truly a massive job—is to work out the vast jigsaw puzzle of fact and circumstances into a complete picture of correct trace element nutrition that everyone can understand and use.

Zinc Influences Circulation

One of the most exciting curative applications of zinc is in the treatment of atherosclerosis (hardening of the arteries). No disease causes more deaths in this country each year. Little by little, as people age, their arteries become partially filled with a soft, pasty, fat-containing material. This limits blood circulation. Hardly anyone is immune to the process of artery hardening, and the result of that clogging is devastating.

William Strain, Ph.D., made an important observation a few years ago about the mineral situation of atherosclerosis victims. He found that all people with that disease in an experimental group of twenty-five unselected male patients had low levels of zinc in their hair. There was no doubt that these people actually had atherosclerosis, because in all cases their

101

arteries had been examined either by surgery or arteriography, a method by which opacifying agents are injected into the arteries and X-ray photographs made. While normal people had 125 to 150 parts per million of zinc in their hair, the atherosclerosis patients had a mean of 62.2 parts per million—less than half of normal.

Other scientists had made the same observation before. B. L. Vallee of Harvard reported in 1956 that heart attack victims had serum zinc levels of sixty-seven parts per million, in comparison with 120 parts per million in normal people. In 1963, Russian scientist N. F. Volkov had also found low zinc levels in seventy-two people suffering from atherosclerosis.

Walter J. Pories, M.D., who had participated in Dr. Strain's original studies as a medical student, decided to try something which had not been done before. He gave large oral doses of zinc to a group of thirty-six patients with advanced atherosclerosis that could not be helped by surgery. For as long as thirty-nine months, these people took 150 milligrams of zinc a day, in the form of zinc sulfate. All had intermittent claudication, a painful condition of the legs caused by the narrowing of the leg arteries as a result of atherosclerosis. There was a remarkable improvement in these people's conditions as a result of the zinc therapy.

Still another link between low zinc levels and heart disease was reported last year by researchers at the University of Cincinnati Medical Center. They found that the higher the dietary intake of zinc and copper (another essential trace element), the lower the level of deposit-forming fats like cholesterol in the blood.

"Perhaps man is particularly vulnerable to increases in cholesterol because he has enough zinc and copper in his body for good growth, but not enough to forestall high and potentially dangerous levels of the blood fat," concluded Dr. Harold G. Petering, one of the researchers.

Dr. Strain and other scientists investigating trace elements are enthusiastic about the promise of relief that zinc therapy holds for victims of hardening of the arteries and other degenerative diseases. "The results are very encouraging," Dr. Strain has said, "since the degenerative diseases become progressively worse and rarely show improvement. Zinc as a means of regulating growth and repair has application from the womb to the tomb."

Leg Ulcers Respond to Zinc Therapy

Although there is probably no magic about the help zinc gives to leg problems, it is interesting that not only the arteries of the legs are improved. Ulcers from poor venous circulation of the legs have healed more rapidly when high-potency zinc supplements are prescribed. The first report we saw of that effect was an article in the October 31, 1970 issue of *The Lancet,* reporting the cures of venous leg ulcers achieved by two British physicians, M. W. Greaves and A. W. Skillen. Later, we discovered that S. L. Husain, a dermatologist in Glasgow, Scotland, had reported earlier in *The Lancet* on a series of leg ulcers healed by zinc sulfate therapy in a controlled study.

Similar results on the healing of leg ulcers by zinc therapy have been published by investigators in Jamaica and Sweden. In Kingston, Jamaica, Serjeant and associates found that zinc therapy promoted the healing of leg ulcers of patients with sickle-cell anemia. Haeger's group in Malmo, Sweden, reported that in controlled studies there was a measurable effect from zinc therapy in healing after the 30th day.

103

Sealing the Connection between Zinc and Healing Power

In the October 14, 1972 issue of *The Lancet,* the Swedish doctors T. Hallböök and E. Lanner from Lund published data showing that zinc therapy was effective especially when the patient was zinc deficient, and that three weeks or longer was needed for a measurable effect. Analyses showed that the zinc levels of the blood rose as the treatment continued. "This points to a definite relation between serum-zinc and healing power," Drs. Hallböök and Lanner said.

The connection between zinc and the healing power of the body is most interesting, and leads to other opportunities for therapy. Of course, it's important to realize that the surface of the subject has just been scratched. Yet it's hard to overlook the implications of studies which show that large numbers of people who are hospitalized for a variety of different diseases have low levels of zinc in their bodies. "Surgical trauma, accidental injury and long bone fractures all cause the body to lose large amounts of zinc in the urine," an article in the October 16, 1972 issue of *The Journal of the American Medical Association* reported. "The cumulative losses are large," said Gordon S. Fell, Ph.D., "and could lead to zinc deficiency in severe cases, indicating that oral or intravenous zinc supplementation might aid the patient."

An even longer list of diseases and health problems connected with low zinc levels is presented by James A. Halsted and J. Cecil Smith, Jr., of the Trace Element Research Laboratory at George Washington University School of Medicine in Washington, D.C. They found low zinc levels in the blood plasma of people suffering from alcoholic cirrhosis, other liver diseases, active tuberculosis, ulcers, uremia, heart attack, pulmonary infection, mongolism, and cystic fibrosis with growth retardation. They also noted that pregnant women as well as women taking oral contraceptives had low levels of zinc in their blood plasma, the body substance they used for measurement. Most interesting of all, they were able to find no illness or conditions that caused the blood plasma to have higher-than-normal levels of zinc. That's quite a powerful indication of the benign nature of this remarkable trace element!

No part of the human anatomy contains more zinc than the prostate. Actually, a healthy man has several times more zinc in his prostate than he does in most other soft tissues of his body. Although much research about the role of trace elements in health and disease remains to be done, it's hard to overlook the importance of zinc to an organ like the prostate when so much of that trace element is present. Also quite significant is the finding that in several types of prostate problems—particularly prostate cancer and chronic abacterial prostatis—the levels of zinc in the prostate gland decline. That effect has been noted by several investigators.

Can large doses of zinc improve prostate health? Yes it can, report Drs. Irving M. Bush and Alfred Zamm and their colleagues at Cook County Hospital in Chicago, a group that has been working for years on the relationship of zinc to the health of the urinary system. Among other things, they found that they can easily find out how much zinc is in the prostate by analyzing samples of semen, the fluid produced by that gland. Their numerous tests have shown that seven percent of men have low levels of zinc in their semen, and thirty percent more are borderline.

Zinc therapy given to men suffering from chronic abacterial prostatis produced good results in seventy percent of forty men in a test group given that treatment. And while getting the zinc, these patients showed a significant increase in the zinc levels of their semen, and hence in their prostate glands.

Does the lower amount of zinc in our diets help to bring on the many medical problems in which low zinc levels have been observed, or is the decline in zinc of the prostate and other parts of the body purely the result of a disease process not associated with nutrition? The final answers are not yet in, but it's apparent that zinc therapy can be used much more widely to improve health at this stage of the development of trace element science.

Why Are Doctors Slow to Use Zinc as a Treatment?

Use of zinc and other trace elements in dealing with disease is rare today in American medical practice. There seems to be a tremendous gap between the remarkable things being discovered in laboratories and at research institutions, and the medical care given by average physicians. Every year, trace element symposiums broadcast reports telling of the importance of minor minerals to health, yet the impact of that information on the minds and methods of doctors is small.

Some medical clinics have made large investments in analytical apparatus, expecting doctors to use trace element science to help diagnose and treat disease. They find that this expensive equipment stands idle much of the time.

Why should doctors be so reluctant to use the benefits that this important new scientific effort can bring to their patients? Here, in outline form, is my opinion:

1. Trace elements are viewed by doctors as pri-

marily a nutritional problem, and nutrition gets very low priority. Like non-swimmers hanging onto a raft, they cling to the now-outdated idea that "Americans are the best-fed people on earth," and that if anyone eats a normal diet he or she is bound to get all the food elements needed. As I pointed out previously, the typical American diet is *causing* zinc deficiency, and is exposing many to serious trace element problems. But most doctors have not yet gotten that message.

2. Trace element science can be used most easily to *prevent* disease, and doctors are oriented too much toward therapy for acute disease. The best approach to real health through trace elements is to take in what you need over a lifetime, through both natural foods and food supplements.

3. Used as a therapy, zinc produces results slowly—perhaps too slowly to interest some doctors. Several studies have shown that even large doses of zinc, taken by mouth, don't produce an effect for several weeks or a month. Since many people tend to stop taking prescribed medications long before their doctors want them to stop, the persistence needed for effective zinc therapy could present an educational problem.

4. Zinc therapy does not use an expensive miracle drug, but a common mineral that is available cheaply in the form of zinc sulfate. Natural forms of zinc are more expensive, but zinc sulfate—the high-potency form now used most widely for therapeutic purposes is very cheap. There is no big profit in selling zinc as a drug, hence no advertising for zinc in medical journals. Many doctors depend on such advertising for both education and inspiration.

5. Perhaps most important of all, many doctors still stick with the wrong idea that, because they can't identify any zinc-deficient people among their

patients, the amount of zinc in the normal American food supply must be adequate. Writing in *World Review of Nutrition and Dietetics* (Vol. 12, 1970) M. R. Spivey Fox of the Food and Drug Administration called that "The most inaccurate means of estimating the human being's need for zinc." She said that way of looking at zinc nutrition "is not founded on adequate scientific data," and "is inaccurate if for no other reason than that the amounts of a nutrient that prevent deficiency symptoms are not necessarily identical with optimal intakes."

Get More Zinc and Keep It

There are a number of things we can do to help insure that we get more than just the marginal amount of zinc that is the norm. And there are things we can do to help keep what zinc we do get. Here are some sugestions:

1. —Eat more sprouted grain. Sprouting neutralizes phytic acid, the chelating agent, naturally present in most grains and seeds, that ties up zinc. When you eat sprouts, you can be sure that your body is using almost all the zinc that's in the food.

2. —Eat some meat and fish. Although values for zinc tend to fluctuate from one sample to the next, meat and fish are routinely richer than other kinds of food. In fact, when you consider the phytate problem in whole grains, vegetarians appear to be inviting zinc deficiency. It's not necessary to go overboard on meat, but eat at least some to help build up your zinc stores.

3. —Drink less alcohol. "The typical American cocktail party is the greatest de-zincer going," says zinc-researcher, Walter J. Pories, M.D. "Alcohol flushes zinc out of the system into the urine," he points out.

4. —Get a sample of your hair tested to find your zinc status.

5. —Take naturally derived zinc supplements. Some such supplements are now on the market, although the potency of zinc they offer is too small. However, because of the growing realization of the vital importance of zinc to good nutrition, there are bound to be improvements soon in the number and quality of zinc supplements sold over-the-counter—without a prescription.

In a recent phone conversation, Dr. Oberleas told me that he recommends the use of a zinc supplement of at least ten milligrams daily dosage, with up to twenty-five milligrams of zinc per day even more desirable. The new Food and Drug Administration Dietary Food Regulations—much attacked because of the low potency limits they impose on most nutrients —at least provide a reference point to consider the zinc problem. The FDA rules say that fifteen milligrams of zinc is the recommended daily allowance. If those rules were to be put into effect as now written, they would allow a maximum of one and one-half times that amount, or 22.5 milligrams of zinc per listed daily dosage of a supplement.

The health-minded public has yet to catch up with even the conservative FDA in the field of zinc supplementation. The only two zinc supplements now on the market that I know about contain a maximum of 1.5 milligrams of zinc per tablet. The labels indicate a daily dosage of four tables per day, providing six milligrams of zinc daily in one case and two milligrams of zinc in the other. Those products are supplying roughly a third or less of the amount of zinc that even the FDA considers reasonable for an over-the-counter food supplement.

Some people are now taking much larger amounts of zinc in supplement form—sometimes going as high as several hundred milligrams a day. However, those supplements are available on prescription only, and their source of zinc is zinc sulfate. That compound has been widely used for research and for treating people who suffer from injuries or diseases which can be helped by drastic increases in zinc intake. The advantage of zinc sulfate as a supplement is that it is inexpensive, and contains a lot of zinc per unit of volume. But it suffers the strong disadvantage of not being natural or naturally derived, in the sense that sulfate breaks down into sulfuric acid in the stomach. Since sulfuric acid is quite corrosive, and is not the kind of acid that the stomach is accustomed to coping with, zinc sulfate is known to cause frequent stomach upset problems in susceptible people. So let's cross off zinc sulfate as a supplement.

It's quite possible that an enterprising maker of food supplements may be able to find sources of oysters and herrings that are sufficiently pure and rich in zinc and concentrate them into food-source zinc supplements. However, the problem is not an easy one, because the trace element content of any food varies, sometimes spectacularly. For example, it's known that oysters growing on the West Coast of the U.S. are not nearly as rich in zinc as oysters plucked from the shores of the East Coast. Why is that? No one knows, but it is the kind of problem that must be faced by anyone marketing a food which is warranted to contain a certain amount of zinc. Ultimately I think that problem will be solved and supplements made directly from high-zinc foods will become available.

Bone meal is worth discussing as a zinc supplement. The zinc content in bone is higher than that of other tissues. There is little or no phytate in bone or other animal tissue, so what zinc you do take in is absorbed. However, the quantity of zinc in bone meal is not large enough to meet the growing need for this useful and safe trace element. The usual beef bone meal tablet contains 20 to 40 micrograms of zinc. So you might have to take as many as 50 tablets of bone meal to get one milligram of zinc.

Zinc gluconate is the naturally-derived source of zinc that has the most potential for supplement use. It is made by combining zinc mined from the earth with an ingredient of food origin—gluconic acid made from potato starch. Zinc gluconate is not an irritant to the stomach or mucous membranes, and has no known pharmacological action other than to supply zinc to the body, which it does very well. Metals in the gluconate form are very readily taken up from the digestive tract. All in all, zinc gluconate fills the bill quite well for a naturally-derived zinc supplement, and you are undoubtedly going to see it more widely used soon.

The only disadvantages of zinc gluconate are that it is a more expensive source of zinc than other compounds, and is also available only in limited quantities. Will the world's stocks of zinc gluconate be adequate to meet the demand for more naturally-processed zinc? That question remains to be answered, although it's likely that more could be manufactured if the demand were there. And perhaps the price would come down if production were increased. Although there is a shortage of zinc ore, the amount needed for food supplement use is a drop in the bucket compared to the mountains of zinc used to make automobile parts, water pipes, and many other industrial products. So we can be sure that there will be enough zinc available to assure an adequate intake of that important element for those who will use supplements or eat zinc-fortified food.

What other sources of zinc are available for food supplement use? Dr. Oberleas believes that zinc carbonate would be suitable. It is a naturally mined product with little or no modification, but suffers the disadvantage of not having a place on the FDA's Generally Recognized as Safe (GRAS) list. Although zinc carbonate has been widely used in animal nutrition for years, it has not gone through the testing process now required for use as a human food ingredient. That would cost several hundred thousand dollars and might or might not result in ultimate FDA acceptance.

Zinc chloride is approved by the FDA as safe for use in food as a mineral supplement, and is another substance recommended for zinc supplementation by Dr. Oberleas. It doesn't quite meet my standards of naturalness, but Dr. Oberleas notes that it is far better than zinc sulfate, which is now rather widely used in drugs. "The chloride ion is natural to the stomach," Dr. Oberleas told me, where it converts into hydrochloric acid, the natural stomach acid which many people are now taking routinely in supplement form anyway. The main advantage of zinc chloride is that it is cheaper than zinc gluconate.

That pretty well sums up the options for zinc supplementation, a subject which I am sure is going to be of growing interest to more people as they become aware of the hazards of low-zinc living and the benefits that can be achieved by getting enough of this mineral. It is important to realize, in considering the different sources of zinc, that zinc itself is a remarkably benign element. Some of the trace elements that we need in small amounts have to be handled carefully in any amount even slightly larger. They have a small margin of safety, even though they are absolutely essential to good health.

TURN THE ENERGY CRISIS INTO A HEALTH BENEFIT 8

We all know plenty about the energy shortage. Newspapers, magazines, radio and TV have all covered the story of the booming demand for fuel and energy. There is little doubt in anyone's mind, after being exposed to all that information, that, as *Fortune* magazine says, "The Energy Joyride Is Over."

For the sake of making sure that you know what we appear to be up against, I will do some reviewing.

First, America is a country of energy drunkards. We comprise 6 percent of the world's population, yet we use about thirty-five percent of the world's energy production. And we keep *doubling* the amount of energy we use every ten years, so you can see that the amount of energy we require for transportation, industrial production, heating, air conditioning, is far more than that used by citizens of other countries.

Second, the amazing expansion of our energy needs is starting to strain our fuel reserves. About 90 percent of the energy we use comes from fossil fuels —coal, oil and gas. They are called fossil because they are the fossilized remains of plants that for one period in the earth's history sprouted, bloomed and died in fantastic abundance. In those primeval swamps, layer upon layer of giant ferns and similar plants grew and died without decaying into humus,

113

but collected the way peat collects in bogs. Later, ocean sediments covered those plant deposits, and they were compressed and processed naturally into the fuels we use today.

Even though the amount of those fossilized fuels remaining under the surface of the earth boggles the imagination, our reserves are not limitless because of the rapid rate at which they are being used. Gas is scarce already. Oil is in critical supply in some areas of the globe, but abundant in other places. However, much of the oil that we use in the U.S., especially in the populous East Coast area, comes from the Near East. Importing that Arab oil strains our dollar reserves and makes us politically dependent on the countries which supply the oil. It is not a healthy situation.

A third aspect of the energy problem has been created by our growing ecological consciousness and environmental awareness. Nuclear power plants, at one time a promised source of almost unlimited power, are coming along very slowly. People are afraid—rightly—of their accident potential and are worried about the problem of storing the atomic wastes, which must be kept safe from floods, earthquakes and man-made disruption for thousands of years. Today, only a tiny fraction of our total power production comes from nuclear plants, and it appears that they won't supply great amounts of power for a long time to come.

Environmental problems also limit our fossil fuel reserves in several ways. For example, we have enough coal to last several hundred years, but people are objecting—again rightly—to the strip-mining process which devastates valuable lands. So although we have the coal, we may not be able to use it economically, because restoring strip-mined lands to their former quality is expensive. Coal is also dirty, creating air pollution problems even when coal-fired power plants are located far from cities. You probably have read about the large coal-fired power plants at Black Mesa, in Arizona, which are spreading clouds of pollutants over four states to produce enough electricity to supply the Los Angeles metropolitan area.

Pollution control itself requires energy, causing more rapid depletion of energy reserves. Cars equipped with emission controls get less mileage than older cars, because energy must be used to operate the air-purifying equipment. So our current push for cleaner air is causing a rapid increase in our already huge demand for oil.

The best evidence of a crunch is the fact that our leaders are now concerned about saving energy as well as finding new sources of power. The Office of Emergency Preparedness, Executive Office of the President, published a staff study on "The Potential for Energy Conservation." It contains many useful ideas that could help us save some of the energy we have been wasting simply because power sources have been so cheap, at least up to now.

For example, many homes are not only overheated, they're also not insulated nearly well enough. With good insulation in all homes, we could reduce the total energy needs of the United States by 5 percent, a remarkable figure. Super-convenient appliances are another source of energy drain. Frost-free refrigerators, for example, use 50 percent more power than conventional refrigerators. Did you realize that? Must you have that extra convenience, or can you defrost your refrigerator once in a while for the sake of saving electricity? Many air conditioners are wasteful of energy also. Experts tell us that use of more efficient air conditioners, which are available, could save as much electricity as would be generated by three power plants as large as the mammoth one at Black Mesa in Arizona. Transportation is the biggest single energy consumer, requiring 25 percent of our total power needs. Jet planes are the most wasteful. Sending people and goods by air uses six times as much power as auto, truck or rail transport. Up to eight percent of U.S. energy needs could be saved if more efficient methods of moving people and things were used.

Cool Homes Can Be Healthful

No one looks forward to running short of heating fuel in the middle of winter, but don't get the panicky feeling that we are completely at the mercy of winter's icy blasts. The fact is that most American homes are overheated, and their occupants could actually benefit in several ways by turning down the thermostat.

First of all, a cool home does not automatically lead to upper respiratory infection. Experiments with human volunteers have shown that people exposed to cold air—even with their feet soaking in ice water—get no more colds when they contact the appropriate viruses than do people in a warm environment.

Yet it is true that there are more cold sufferers in the winter and late spring than at other times of the year. No one knows for sure why that happens, but statistical studies have shown that the incidence of colds increases shortly after a cold front passes through an area. No amount of home heating is likely to change that fact.

Actually, some experts think that overheating of homes and public buildings is one of the root causes of the surge in colds and related diseases in the winter. There are two theories backing up that assumption:

Warm air is normally much drier than cold air. Add to that condition the drying effect of heating, and you have a household environment where the air is sometimes drier than the Sahara Desert. That causes nasal discomfort, and possibly exposes people to additional risk of sickness.

The belief that colds spread faster in winter because people congregate in heated buildings is generally accepted. The urge to "get in out of the cold" crowds people together. The result is more opportunity for cold germs to spread from one person to another.

A home heated to perhaps sixty-five to sixty-eight degrees can be as healthful (or more healthful) than one kept in the seventies. Moreover, turning down the thermostat only three degrees will save nine percent on fuel. If everyone would do that, existing fuel stocks might be adequate for all our needs.

The body itself is a "heating element" that can be put to effective use to create its own comfortable environment. Here are some suggestions for ways to live well in winter while saving on fuel in your home:

Change the way you dress. One extra layer of soft wool on your body can have a remarkable insulating effect. I was in Northern China in January and February of 1973 and I saw that the Chinese get along very well in their cool homes by wearing sweaters both on their upper and lower body. They wear cotton underwear and a heavy cotton suit over the sweater. Sometimes even cotton padding is used. Such clothing is very comfortable.

Pay special attention to keeping your feet warm, even indoors. Many people who would be satisfied with a cooler general temperature in their homes, are sensitive to cold drafts around the floor. That problem can be corrected by careful insulating and weather-stripping, or simply by investing in a pair of down-filled bootees. They are readily available at a sporting-goods store or from a company selling clothing for hikers and mountain climbers. These down-filled socks are meant to be used inside boots, but they're extremely comfortable for lounging indoors on cold, winter evenings.

Use a down or dacron comforter on your bed. It will keep you plenty warm at night, even in a cold room. Outdoorsmen who know how to protect themselves against the wind use down sleeping bags and sleep comfortably in below-zero temperatures. So allowing the bedroom temperature to drop into the 50's should present no challenge at all.

Consider a nutritional approach to withstanding cold. "Low temperatures increase our need for vitamin C, and beneficial effects of ascorbic acid have been observed in people exposed to extremely low temperatures," says Dr. Marie-Louis Desbarets-Schonbaum, assistant professor of pharmacology at the University of Toronto.

"People exposed to chilly temperatures and whose food supply was limited have been found to develop disturbances in the circulation of their feet," she said. "Such problems could be relieved or avoided if those people were given extra ascorbic acid." How the vitamin C effect works is still a mystery, but Dr. Schonbaum believes that vitamin C stimulates enzyme activity, which in turn affects blood circulation.

Other experiments done in Canada more than ten years ago by biologist Louis-Paul Dugal of the University of Ottawa revealed that monkeys given large amounts of vitamin C were able to withstand cold better than other monkeys. He attributed his results to stimulation of production of thyroid and medullary hormones.

One side benefit of keeping your home cooler in the winter could be liberating yourself from the belief that the only place to be warm and comfortable during cold weather is indoors. If your home temperature is kept closer to that outside—and you conserve body heat with proper indoor clothing—you won't feel as great a shock when you venture out.

Your urge to exercise will also be stimulated—and movement is the greatest warmer-upper of all. Cross-country skiers, for example, spend hours outside during winter while wearing a thin jacket or shirt, and if anything they're overheated. But they keep moving constantly, radiating large amounts of heat from their bodies.

Of course, constant movement is no answer to the problem of keeping comfortably warm indoors a whole winter. But the powerful effect of brisk movement serves to show how effective our personal heat engine is—and how much energy we can save by using it more sensibly.

Energy Shortages Affect Our Food and Health

Americans are such heavy users of energy in all forms that every aspect of our industrialized society is going to be influenced—not only the temperature of our homes in winter, but also the kind and quality of food we eat and the kind of health we enjoy.

Much of our food is transported long distances, for example, especially during the winter months. With food shortages and rising costs, there is going to have to be more emphasis on locally-grown foods and storage of food produced nearby for later consumption.

Even though grain prices are going up as rapidly as the prices of more glamorous foods, we may find ourselves eating more food made with rice, beans, wheat, barley and oats. These foods are efficient converters of free solar energy into carbohydrates and protein, through photosynthesis. Their production consumes much less fossil fuel energy than other kinds of food, so prices are likely to stay within the reach of even limited budgets.

Foods that come wrapped in paper and are highly processed will rise in price faster than other kinds of food, as energy prices rise. For example, the way food is served in many fast-food restaurants is wasteful of energy.

Engineering professor Bruce M. Hannon of the University of Illinois computed that the McDonald's chain of restaurants alone used up the energy equivalent of 12.7 million tons of coal in 1972. "That's enough energy to keep the cities of Pittsburgh, Boston, Washington and San Francisco supplied with electric power for the entire year," he said. Fast-food restaurants consume so much power because their serving dishes, utensils, wrappers, and so forth are all one-way. They aren't reused, like dishes at home.

It's in the area of health and fitness that the energy crisis is certain to have its most dramatic and prompt effect. We have grown accustomed to having fuel-powered machines do work for us, instead of using our own muscles. As a result, Americans are now flabbier than ever.

Most people could soon strengthen their leg muscles sufficiently to be able to walk short distances instead of taking their car. But other tasks might prove too strenuous for aging joints and muscles that have not been kept in condition by regular use. For example, could you still push a hand mower around your large lawn, if gasoline shortages forced you to try?

Even more critical is the direct health risk that might result from cutbacks in air conditioning. High heat and humidity put extra stress on older and sickly people. Many such people in our society today are nearly as dependent on air conditioning as some polio victims are on their iron lungs.

Dr. George E. Burch, chairman of the Department of Medicine at Tulane University Medical School, is one physician who is convinced that air conditioning keeps some people alive. "In congestive heart failure, air conditioning is more important than oxygen," he says.

Are we going to have to give up air conditioning because of energy shortages? Probably not entirely, but we may have to cut back by keeping homes, cars and public buildings at slightly higher temperatures in summer. That could cause a marginal, but still measurable, effect on the health of chronically sick people.

If you're concerned about these possible results of energy restrictions, act now.

Start to improve your fitness gradually. There's no question that people who are physically fit will be better able to cope with the demands that a lowered use of energy is going to make on our bodies. Walking is the best exercise of all, especially for people who have weakened themselves by decades of riding. It builds up not only the legs and thighs, but the lungs as well if the walks are brisk.

Get your weight down. Added pounds aggravate the stress and strain of living with summer's heat, and also makes exercise more work. So make eating less part of your personal program to get in shape for low-energy living.

Do more gardening if you have the land available. There's no question that food produced in your own garden makes a lower demand on energy reserves than food grown on large farms and shipped long distances.

Get used to living without air conditioning whenever possible, to prepare for possible future emergency situations. Air conditioning is a tremendous drain on our energy reserves. In fact, the 200 million people in the U.S. use as much energy for air conditioning as all 800 million people in China use for *all their power requirements.*

The Good Life through Less Gasoline

Many Americans react as strongly to the prospect of automobile fuel shortages as they do to the thought of a cut-back in home-heating fuels. Are you prepared for life with less gasoline?

Gasoline rationing isn't necessarily the end of the world. More than half the auto trips we make now probably aren't absolutely necessary. Much weekend cruising around, for example, is an aimless quest for mobility and greener pastures. Even without gas rationing, a growing minority of thoughtful people are discovering that it makes more sense to plan activities carefully to limit the need to drive. They have some compelling reasons and I present them for your consideration.

Pleasure trips sometimes turn into tragedy. "We have almost stopped wincing at the statistics," says John Jerome, former editor of *Car and Driver* magazine. "Almost sixty thousand deaths per year, more than a thousand a week killed, ten thousand a day injured, a billion dollars a month in economic loss."

The present system of auto insurance is leading us into "a morass of hardships," Senator Frank Moss has charged. "Should more than one car be involved in an accident—the tug and haul begins," he said. "Whose fault was it? Who has insurance and who does not? If both are insured, whose company should pay? Sometimes it is months—even years—before opposing attorneys or the courts decide."

While clogging our roads and choking our lungs, cars "gobble natural resources like cocktail peanuts," Jerome notes in his book, *The Death of the Automobile* (Norton).

What alternatives are there to such endless roaming? Actually, right in your own yard or immediate neighborhood there are scores of ways to fill leisure time with rewarding activity: Start gardening, relearn the art of conversation and fellowship, develop a skill or learn a craft, learn to play a musical instrument, master a second language.

No matter how you choose to do it, severing your leisure-time dependence on the automobile will simplify your life and give you a head start toward a lifestyle we may all share someday. As Jerome puts it, "Every day new elements click into place: the risk, the cost, the delay, the bother, the crowding and congestion. The rage. When the destination diminishes as the task of getting there grows, when the endless prospect of unrelieved blight conquers the remaining vistas, when no conceivable *place* holds any hope of being different from any other . . . then we will stay home."

Will Mass-Transit Save Us?

For years, we've been hearing that the only way to save ourselves from increasing urban congestion is a better mass transit system. Convince people to leave their cars at home, and things will flow smoothly, the planners say.

But all the new buses, trains, monorails and subways in the world may not be enough to keep the cities from choking. New transit lines spur more development, generating more movement and more crowding. Ultimately, we reach a limit to the number of people who can be transported in a given area.

"There is growing evidence that rapid transit may be no more successful than express highways in satisfactorily solving traffic congestion," writes Wilfred Owen in his book, *The Accessible City.* If Owen is right and the planners are wrong, we're all going to be in trouble—unless we start walking. What is needed, he says, is a whole new approach to urban design that puts living, shopping and working facilities all *within walking distance.*

Walking has always been the most reliable and least polluting mode of transit. Many of Europe's cities have no mass transportation method because nearly everything is within walking distance. Those cities are among the most pleasant places in the world to live.

Walking is the only method of transportation in most Chinese villages and towns, according to Dr. Ernst Winter, environmental consultant to the U.N. There are no streets or roads through the towns, only foot paths. Many villages are connected to other communities by canals. In the back country, dirt roads connect towns. But they end at the village gates. Animals and carts are left at the outskirts of the town, and goods are carried into homes on peoples' shoulders. That permits quiet access to homes, and pleasant living conditions. The only way that the Chinese can live happily in such close, over-populated conditions is by being extra careful and considerate of the feelings of others.

The current Chinese regime is firmly against auto ownership, and promotes cycling and walking

instead. Foot and cycle traffic is directed by police—
or by anyone.

In the United States, walking has been designed
out of new developments and even in cities, our over-
taxed transportation networks suffer, and so does our
health. As our cities become clogged with stalled
transport, our bodies become flabby and weak. In re-
structuring cities, we can also promote fitness by de-
signing some necessary walking into transportation
plans, for even short walks can do wonders for health
and disposition.

If You're Riding, Use a Bicycle

If you're riding at all, current conditions make
it clear that there's no way to go but up for the bicycle! In fact, a dramatic growth in the number of
bicycles and cyclists is a certainty, and bicycle sales
outlets are bound to increase in number too.

Bicycle sales are booming because they satisfy
growing needs. Recreation is in big demand, and
bikes are fun to ride. Building physical fitness is a
problem for many, and bicycle riding is good exercise.

Bicycles get you around fast, at low cost. Pollution control is also imperative. Nothing beats the
bicycle as an example of pollution-free technology.

Bicycles have been popular before, especially
during the great American bicycle fad around the
turn of the century. This time the attraction for the
bicycle is likely to stick because we need it.

Even the federal government recognizes that bicycles are now a "viable mode of transportation."
The Department of Transportation held a two-day
"Bicycles—U.S.A." conference in Cambridge, Massachusetts to help two-wheelers find their "rightful
place in the multi-modal mix," repeating the words

of Assistant Secretary of Transportation John E. Hirten.

In plain English, that means bicycles are here to stay, but we have to find some way for pedal power to coexist peacefully with piston power. For the new and booming popularity of the cycle is not without its problems.

Safety is the main concern. A man on a bicycle is simply no match for the typical overpowered motorist, who wears his car as armor and often moves too fast to see a bicyclist until a collision is inevitable. In California, where bicycles are really "in," a safety expert has predicted that 25,000 cyclists will be killed or injured in that state alone during 1975.

The safety issue is behind the growing demand for special bicycle paths and "bikeways." Regular roads and highways are hazardous places to ride bicycles, and they're getting more dangerous as the number of cyclists and drivers increases.

Some of the more dedicated cyclists aren't happy about the thought of being segregated on special paths. They see nothing wrong with regular roads as conduits for bicycles from one place to another, and think that motorists should be forced to reduce speed and otherwise accommodate to growing bicycle traffic.

That militant spirit has already produced results in some cities. New York's Central Park is closed to automobiles on Saturdays and Sundays, so the bicyclists can have free rein. Also, bicycle lanes have been painted on streets in some towns, forcing autos to give up part of the road to pedalers.

The fuel shortage is pushing public opinion toward the cyclists' point of view; it almost insures that two-wheelers are going to continue to make inroads on the road.

Do you want to become part of the bicycle movement? Here are some ideas that will help in making the transition.

1. Be aware that bicycles are made in different sizes to fit the varying body conformations. Also, different types of cycles are useful for different purposes. If you're a novice to cycling, seek out a dealer who is interested in fitting you with the proper machine for your personal needs.

2. Start riding slowly and carefully, building up your tolerance for exercise gradually. Bicycle-riding can be a strain on legs and lungs weakened by a sedentary life.

3. Follow safety rules. Avoid riding at night. Even with lights and reflectors it is dangerous. Wear bright-colored clothes whenever you ride, so automobile drivers can see you easily. Mount a high-flying pennant on your bike for added visibility. And even if you have the right-of-way at an intersection, move cautiously because auto drivers may not see you.

4. Dress properly and you can ride in all seasons. Only the most severe blizzards force some northern bicycle commuters to take to the bus. Warm boots and gloves are a necessity, but the exercise of cycling soon warms you up inside even if you are wearing a light jacket.

5. Learn how to lubricate and adjust your machine. The popular 10-speed bikes are easy to ride and a pleasure to own, but they need attention to stay in top shape. Periodic oiling will keep the gear mechanism and chain working longer, and will help avoid miscues in shifting that could prove dangerous on crowded streets.

6. Buy a good strong chain lock to protect your bicycle when it's parked. As bicycles become more desirable to more and more people, thefts are bound to become even more common.

Will Energy Shortages Cripple Conventional Agriculture?

Most of the commentaries carefully document the role of energy in home-heating, in industry and in transportation, but fail to mention the extremely important role that cultivation of the soil plays in the whole power equation. In typical human fashion, people think only about the most visible and apparent power sources. They overlook the fact that green plants are the vital link that enables us to convert sun energy into food energy, and are far more important to our well-being than coal, oil or gas.

Agriculture, in fact, is the original technique that man used to harness power to fuel an expanding economy. Plants have their roots in the almost inexhaustible mineral resources of the earth's crust, and their leaves are exposed to both the useful gases of the atmosphere (carbon dioxide is the gas plants needs most) and to the rays of the sun.

Through the remarkable process of photosynthesis, all these useful things are converted into carbohydrates, the food energy without which we could not survive. It's a remarkably simple and efficient process. And if it's handled right, photosynthesis is not only a non-polluting power source, but is constructively beneficial to the environment. The organic matter created by photosynthesis converts naturally into humus, improving the fertility of the soil. And the stored harvests of argiculture are just as much energy resources as are deposits of coal, or the charge of an electric battery.

The more organic a farming or gardening system is, the more efficient is the energy yield of that enterprise. And by the same token, the more high-powered, technological and agribusiness-oriented agriculture becomes, the less efficient is its yield of food energy—in relation to power consumed. No coal, oil or gas was needed to run an old-time farm. Homes were heated with wood, from trees grown right on the farm. Agriculture used to be entirely self-contained, from an energy standpoint. Organic cultivation is more efficient because a greater proportion of its energy input comes from sun energy, which is free. Organic cultivation of the soil also is carried on to a large extent by human hands, aided with power equipment but not with the massive inputs of potent synthetic fertilizers and pesticides. Those chemical tools are made with the use of large amounts of fossil fuel energy. So when farmers and gardeners put synthetic materials on their land, they are in effect consuming the same kind of energy that powers automobiles and industrial plants, and air-conditions homes.

We don't yet know exactly how much more efficient organic growing is than conventional growing, from the point of view of energy consumption. But we do know that conventional agriculture—at least as carried on in the U.S.—is no longer an energy-producing segment of our economy.

The power for large farm machines—which replace the many millions of farm workers now living in cities—also comes from stored energy sources. When farming was done with horses, the animals' feed was grown right on the farm. Now farmers import tractor fuel, and pay high prices for it. Tractor fuel alone, without considering the energy needed to produce and transport synthetic fertilizers and pesticides, is about equal to the total energy yield of agriculture. That information comes from the excellent article "Farming with Petroleum," by Michael J. Perelman in the October 1972 issue of *Environment*.

The main purpose of Perelman's article is to point out that American agriculture should not be cited for efficiency just because it can produce a lot of food with only a little human help. He cites as misleading the statement by Clifford Hardin, former Secretary of Agriculture, that "One man can take care of 60,000 to 75,000 chickens, 5,000 feedlot cattle, or 50 to 60 milk cows."

"After all," says Perelman, "no man alive can really feed 75,000 chickens by himself. In reality he is aided by many other men who make equipment and other necessities for raising chickens, even though some of them might never set foot on a farm." And all of those other men are consuming energy, and the products they create consume energy too when they are used on the farm. So even though our mechanized farms give the impression of tremendous efficiency, they are buying that efficiency with cheap fuel. *As the price of that fuel goes up, or as it becomes so scarce as to be unavailable, the inadequate energy yields of conventional farms will be exposed.*

And as the price of fuel goes up, more people are going to turn to gardening and small-scale farming as ways to produce needed food energy. There is plenty of evidence that human activity, especially when applied to making things grow in the soil, is a fantastically rewarding way to capture the energy of the sun and convert it into useful power. In his *Environment* article, Perelman cites the energy productivity of Chinese paddy culture of rice, which is so dependent on human labor that it really qualifies as a form of large-scale gardening. Chinese wet rice agriculture, says Perelman, can produce 53.5 British thermal units of energy for each BTU of human energy used in farming it. That means that for each unit of energy the farmer expends, he gets back over 50 in return.

By contrast, conventional agriculture returns only about one-fifth of a BTU in the form of food energy for each unit of fossil fuel that is expended in plowing, cultivation, harvesting and storing crops. Looked at in that way, we can see that our vaunted agricultural productivity is extremely vulnerable to energy shortages, and is not nearly as rewarding per unit of energy expended as more primitive types of farming.

The trend toward organic, chemical-free agriculture is being hampered by voices from the agribusiness camp saying that fifty million Americans will starve if farmers return to natural methods. Many people believe those claims, despite the fact that they are made by people with a vested interest in the sale of artificial fertilizers and pesticides.

Taking an objective look at the issues of organic versus chemical agriculture is difficult, because almost everyone is on either one side or the other. Also, the issues are complex. For example, large-scale movements of people from cities back to farms would have to take place to provide the manpower for an organic agriculture.

Perhaps you can now see the precarious position that conventional agriculture is in. Fossil fuels won't last forever. They may not last for more than another few generations, at growing rates of use. Waiting for the sun to make more coal and oil is out of the question. We don't have the time, and geographical conditions aren't right.

Although the sun shining on farms today still supplies a large amount of the total energy used, the proportion coming from fossil fuels is vital to the operation of the modern farming system. Take away coal, oil and gas and many more than fifty million people would starve.

Most concern about possible energy shortages is focused on more visible and obvious energy consumption than agriculture. Farm use of power should get far more consideration.

Efforts to recycle garbage and sewage as fertilizer should be intensified, because they are wasted power sources. Biological control of insects, which uses less fossil-fuel power than chemical pesticides, should be emphasized.

Since tractors and other farm machines can run only on oil or gas, those fuels should be conserved for that purpose. All energy input of farms should be examined, and the least efficient restricted. We have to remember that farms are places to maximize photosynthesis, and that the energy of the sun is free. The sun will be here long after coal, oil and gas are exhausted.

Farmers must plant more cover crops to catch the sun's rays during all seasons of the year. Bare ground means sun energy is being wasted. Cover crops convert soil minerals to organic compounds that improve soil fertility for use in future years.

Movement of people away from the land must be reversed by creating more opportunities for re-populating the countryside. Sun-powered agriculture needs people on the land to make it work. There should be more vegetable gardening, for example. One person cultivating a couple of acres can help convert large amounts of sun energy into food, in a garden.

Transportation of food from one part of the country to another should be limited. Fossil fuel used for movement of food would be saved, and localized agriculture would be encouraged.

The real issue in feeding the world is not whether organic or chemical methods are the most productive, but are we making the best possible use of our limited power sources?

The Chinese have the most effective organic farming program on the face of the earth. Sewage, garbage and crop wastes are not piled in landfills, dumped into rivers or burned in China. They are quickly returned to the soil to help keep it fertile. Land stays productive for thousands of years, and large families are supported on only a few acres.

An American soil scientist, Dr. F. H. King, documented the unique workings of Chinese ecology over sixty years ago, in his classic book *Farmers of Forty Centuries.* King traveled extensively through the Orient, observing with his trained eye how Chinese practices of saving and using everything differed so much from our wasteful way of life.

The exact procedure for making compost was reported by King, former head of the U.S. Department of Agriculture Division of Soil Management. He learned how Chinese engineers refused to dump human wastes into rivers, even in large cities. They sold the wastes to farmers.

Sir Albert Howard, the English scientist who pioneered organic farming, was greatly influenced by King's insights. Many aspects of Chinese gardening, farming and even diet were incorporated into Howard's no-chemical system.

The flow of ecology ideas from the East didn't stop there. Oriental culture has been a constant source of ideas for people seeking alternative life styles, and a more varied natural-food diet.

Free Energy Is Available

Although the Chinese appear to be functioning quite well on the limited fuel supplies, the energy picture for us isn't a bright one. True, researchers around the globe are trying to tap totally new sources of energy. We read about breeder reactors that make their own atomic fuel, controlled fusion reactions that will release fantastic amounts of energy, plus a variety of other energy sources including geothermal plants that will tap the heat of the earth's molten core.

Don't expect any of those energy alternatives to make a big contribution to the massive power demands of the American economy in the near future, however. All of them are technologically sophisticated, and will require plenty of both time and good luck to be perfected. Remember how long it has taken for nuclear power to even begin to fulfill its promise of cheap energy. There's a good chance that the other new energy sources that are now promised will also prove to be disappointing. Our present high-energy civilization is based on simply lifting coal and oil from the earth and using it as concentrated power sources. No other kind of new energy promises to be nearly that easy to use.

As the ecologists say, there's no such thing as a free lunch. But there are sources of free energy, and the rush to find and develop them makes the Gold Rush of 1849 look like a stroll in the park by comparison.

Hundreds of scientists and backyard inventors are working overtime in a race for low-cost, alternate energy sources. Anyone observing the birth of this new energy industry can't help noticing important ways it is different from the mining and oil-pumping efforts of the past, however. That word "free" is treated importantly, even reverently. Not only are inventors hoping to show people how to capture their own energy at no cost (or at least at very little expense), but they're aiming to free people from domination by corporations and countries sitting on large stockpiles of conventional energy.

Surprisingly, there are quite a few energy sources suitable for such low-cost development. Some have been used before, others represent brand-new ideas, but almost all are bound to increase in popularity in years to come.

People power is getting new attention. The human body can produce a remarkable output of movement power and heat energy from a diet of ordinary food.

Several firms are already marketing lightweight, enclosed two-seater people-powered vehicles that are propelled by pedaling, instead of by internal combustion engines. Users report they are easy to handle and accelerate, thanks to a sophisticated gearing system.

With the addition of a flywheel, these vehicles could become stationary power sources charging batteries that would operate small refrigerators and freezers intermittently. Future power blackouts may start people pedaling away to save their frozen foods.

Animal wastes can produce methane gas. Families in Taiwan are cooking with a fuel that goes to waste in more affluent countries—natural methane gas generated by hog manure. And no one is holding his nose! The pig methane is reportedly simple, reliable, economical and clean.

Bubbles that rise in a liquid hog manure are more than fifty percent methane, a colorless, odorless, flammable hydrocarbon produced when organic matter decomposes. A steel box inverted over the manure captures the gas, and a plastic tube feeds it from the pig pen to a kitchen burner. Similar systems, utilizing the wastes from cattle and other livestock, are being developed in western countries.

Many students of alternate power sources are getting excited about capturing the energy of the wind. Up to now, the big stumbling block has been what to do on days the wind doesn't blow. But new developments in storage battery systems could solve that problem. And windmills with variable pitch and self-feathering propellers that can handle any kind of breeze are being developed.

Practical ways to convert the sun's rays into heat and electricity are making possible a new generation of "solar homes." One already-functioning house at the University of Delaware is designed to manufacture eighty percent of its own energy.

Electricity produced by solar cells in the roof is conducted to home appliances such as the electric range, with the excess going to storage batteries for later use.

An engine that takes its power from ocean waves has been tested at the Scripps Institute of Oceanography. It might someday be used to generate power for small coastal communities.

Although not an energy producer, a system of oil toilets developed by Chrysler Corporation could ultimately be a big help in saving precious natural resources. Mineral oil is used instead of water as a flushing and transport medium. As the wastes are filtered out, the oil is recycled and used again and again. According to Chrysler, conventional toilet facilities could easily be converted to this oil system.

By prudently harvesting waste wood from their land, some property owners are assuring themselves of a cheap fuel, independent of utility companies. "A large enough woodlot will supply you with enough wood to heat your house" says *Organic Gardening and Farming* editor Jeff Cox, "and nature will grow back each year what you've taken."

Many more alternate energy sources are waiting to be tapped and perfected. All that is needed is ingenuity and a healthy respect for the environment.

To sum up, there are two ways to avoid the power crunch organically. First, we must start conserving energy by using common sense. Better insulation of our homes is extremely important, and if you think of the word organic in a broad sense that is an organic technique. We must do more walking, especially around cities and towns, and less riding in automobiles. That certainly is organic.

And in deciding to do those things, we must not think that our little effort to conserve is meaningless when compared to the total picture of our energy-hungry civilization. Charles Lindberg gives some advice on that point in his article "Lessons from the Primitive" in *The Reader's Digest*.

"Are we ready to moderate sufficiently our worship of bigness, power, speed and affluence?" he asks. "Can we relearn the values of simplicity, tranquility and balance? Are we bound to our technologies as an addict is bound to drugs, or can we follow a course of action based on human welfare? The answer must come from individuals like you and me, for civilization, with its governments and establishments, is shaped by the forces of human desire."

Finally and just as important, we must learn the energy lessons that agriculture and gardening can teach us. For I am sure that when the energy crunch does hit in full force, the home garden, the home storage shed for food, and the small orchard are going to be widely recognized as more important (and more liberating) energy sources than the ultra-high-technology generating plants now being worked on by researchers. We know that a good garden can yield plenty of storable energy with a moderate amount of work. By comparison, those fancy new power plants are just pipe dreams.

You Must Help Yourself to Better Health 9

The demarcation between life and death is becoming fuzzy. For example, there is no longer a rigid rule that says if your heart stops beating you are dead. I know of at least one case where a supposedly dead person started talking on the operating table—while his heart was being removed for transplanting. The medical people are embarrassed by that sort of thing, and are developing more certain means of determining death.

The brain is now the focus of attention as the last place from which life leaves the body. If your brain is still making waves, you are safe from the transplant surgeon's knife, provided your local hospital subscribes to the right code of ethics. On the surface, the brain wave idea seems like the best way for the medical people to define life and death.

Brain waves are only part of the story of being alive. Many people meet all the medical criteria for aliveness, yet they still feel partly dead. They don't get exhilarated, they don't enjoy anything as much as they used to, and their lives are routine.

What has happened is that life has become mechanized. Technology is everywhere and appears to be the most powerful force in our society. Almost every task that people have to perform or enjoy performing is being taken over by machines. The aims of mechanization are to save labor, lower the cost of production, make life more comfortable, reduce risk of accidents, and to avoid annoying problems of all sorts. All well and good, but what has been overlooked is that mechanization may eventually go so far that people will wonder whether they are needed or not. Don't laugh! Machines have been making machines for a long time—and perhaps we are too far along the road to the *Brave New World* to stop the process.

To understand and cope with this technological world, we must understand and appreciate the idea of partial death. We see evidence all around us of the lingering kind of death that afflicted the dinosaurs. They were obsolete and doomed long before the last member of the clan folded its giant tent and slipped into the muck. Some American institutions are dead but they keep functioning. Magazine experts now believe that the old *Saturday Evening Post* was moribund five years before its last issue appeared, but the presses kept clicking away all that time.

People are the same way. They die by degrees, and such partial death is not always related to age. I know some people in their 70's who have more feeling of being alive, more sheer pleasure of living, than many men and women in their twenties.

The easiest way to slip into the quicksand of partial death is always to seek comfort and security. That is the siren song of technology: buy this little box that plays music and you'll always have a friend; take this drug and you'll always feel high; buy this car and you'll never have to walk. Following that route, our home environment eventually becomes a concentration camp—a comfortable, velvet-lined prison.

Can You Shun Comfort Temporarily?

The first way to find out if you are still fully alive is to ask yourself whether you regularly take some physical and mental risks. Do you think that only crazy people climb mountains, ride horses in jumping races, or ski down tree-lined, rock-studded slopes? If you do, that's a bad sign, because people who do those things have the greatest feeling of aliveness that it's possible to have.

"Man has a need for well-calculated risk on a physical and mental basis," says Sol Roy Rosenthal, M.D., Ph.D., and he ought to know. Dr. Rosenthal is medical director of the Research Foundation in Chicago and a professor of preventive medicine at the University of Illinois. The study of the life-stimulating effect of what he calls Risk Exercise is Dr. Rosenthal's special interest. "Risk is necessary for our daily well-being," he says, and backs up that conclusion with careful study and reflection.

"Risk exercise is the modern counterpart of what our ancestors were confronted with in their everyday lives," he points out in an article in *The Maryland Horse*. "The acts for protection, the maintenance of territorial rights, the foraging for food were some of the daily risks taken for self-preservation. The daily challenges were no foolhardy risks, but were well calculated.

"Undoubtedly, these calculated risks contributed to the molding of our evolution."

In other words, when we stop doing things that require us to stretch our physical and mental resources, to push ourselves a little beyond the point where we are completely safe, we are being unnatu-

141

ral in terms of our historical, human heritage. The part of our soul that used to be exercised by those risks begins to wither, and we start dying.

Of course, the degree of risk necessary to awaken what might be called the risk reflex varies with the need and personality of the individual. James Michener, author of *South Pacific*, stood in the street in Pamplona, Spain, and watched wild bulls rush by a few inches from his gut—just to get the feeling of what it's like to be really alive. On the other hand, a person confined to a wheelchair who learns to stand and walk a few feet is taking a similar kind of risk, for him, and gets the same feeling. The trouble is that the average person thinks running with bulls is too extreme, and he isn't confined to a wheelchair either, so he follows a comfortable middle course, always looking for the safest way. No wonder he feels that something is missing from his life.

Let's examine the kind of risk I mean. Mountain climbing is thought to be a very risky sport, but when practiced by people who are properly trained and equipped climbing is little more dangerous than driving a car. Yet the psychic rewards are far greater. Several summers ago my son David and I took a brief lesson in rock-climbing in the Grand Tetons of Wyoming, and that afternoon, while I was strugling to get up a 200-foot cliff, I wondered continuously what the devil I was doing there. I was pinned solidly to the rock by ropes and pitons, and therefore I was safe, but I certainly didn't *feel* safe.

After the climb I felt an overwhelming relief that the ordeal was over. But mingled with that feeling of relief was an even stronger feeling of happiness at being alive and of walking on solid ground—a feeling of aliveness that surpassed anything I had felt for a long time. The memory of the ordeal fades quickly in my mind, but the pleasure that followed remains. Some day I will probably climb another cliff—maybe several.

The two men who recently climbed the 2,000-foot Wall of the Morning Light on El Capitan were thought by many people to be crazy to try such a climb, and they themselves admitted to a slight touch of insanity. The younger climber, Dean Caldwell, dropped a note when they were half-way up the cliff saying "We must be the most miserable, wet, cold, stinking wretches imaginable." Of course they were. "But we're alive, really alive, like people seldom are," he added.

Too Many of Us Never Do Anything

Do you have to be crazy to be alive? The article on risk exercise in *The Maryland Horse* starts out with the statement that "Some people do the craziest things. . . But too many of us never do anything." If you are in that last category, you should worry about the kind of brain waves you are making, and should start looking around for a few mild risks. Don't cross out of your mind the possibility of doing things that seem a little crazy. After all, so many people are trying to be safe (and are finding that safety dull and boring) that any different way of passing the time is bound to be branded as oddball.

The second method of finding out whether you are really alive is to ask yourself whether you are getting your daily dose of environmental ecstasy. Do you see something each day which causes you to wonder at the beauty of nature—a clear sunset, a clean stream, an unusual bird, animal or flower that requires a high grade, pure environment? Do you have the compulsion to observe, to seek out new things, which would cause you to find intense pleasure in the routine places you pass in your daily life?

Maurice Broun, a naturalist who lives in New Ringgold, Pennsylvania, gives a wonderful lecture, illustrated with slides, which he calls *Environmental Ecstasy*. By getting his camera very close to common, ordinary plants, he shows their remarkable and beautiful structure, invisible when viewed with the naked eye. He arouses in his audience a desire to observe the world more closely, to see beauty where beauty is normally overlooked.

Of course, many people today live where there is little opportunity to see natural things, and to experience environmental ecstasy. But far more people make no effort to sense and enjoy that which is near at hand. One of the spots Maurice Broun is most ecstatic about is the Pine Barrens of New Jersey, which is only a short drive from New York and Philadelphia. Liberally spotted with rare plants, clear streams, and native animals, it is largely ignored by the millions of people living nearby.

We must seek out our daily dose of environmental ecstasy.

Technology is taking from us and giving to machines the fun of making things that are used in everyday life. Have you held in your hand recently anything that was hand made? Probably not. Only a few generations ago, everything that helped people to be more civilized was made by hand—from blankets and dishes to wheels and ax handles. Today, all our utensils are stamped from molds, and they stir in our minds the vision of some clever machine turning out dishes and knives and forks rather than the knowledge that other human hands can help us live a better life. As a result, we have become less human, less alive.

We lose aliveness also because we are forgetting the craft skills that helped us create a way of life from natural raw materials. Who today knows how to dig a well, make a wooden bowl, weave cloth, or pluck a chicken? Not many modern people know these things; instead they have the specialized knowledge to run computers and tend automatic machines. However, there is a growing revival of old-time craft skills among people who know the feeling of aliveness that creating can give. As hobbies, rather than out of necessity, people are gardening, making pottery, doing silverwork, and even making candles. That kind of skill gives a feeling of completeness to life that goes far beyond the dollars-and-cents value of what you create. If you can see and feel something that you have made yourself, you get a greater sense of your own usefulness, and aliveness.

All three of these standards for judging your aliveness—risk, ecstasy, creation—are tied together by the question of who really is in charge here, people or machines? Yes, it is very easy to allow machines to do more of our work, but to the extent that this happens we give up more of the sense of being alive.

Why Is Self-Diagnosis a Dirty Word?

While we may not be able to hold back what passes for progress on the grand scale, we can still create, in our own lives, islands of vitality. More than that, we can resolve to keep careful watch on our bodies, to know when we have a firm hold on good health and to recognize the first sign that it is beginning to slip from our grasp and what is wrong.

Self-diagnosis is a dirty word to many doctors and other health workers. They are convinced that average people don't have the ability to figure out their own health problems, and should always seek professional help.

145

There's some merit to those concerns. Doctors are notoriously prone to misdiagnose their own health problems, so how can untrained laymen figure out what's wrong with themselves? Of course, if the self-diagnosis is wrong, the self-treatment is likely to be wrong too, and that can lead to more serious problems.

However, a certain amount of self-diagnosis is necessary. Everyone must take some responsibility for his own health, and handle minor problems like bumps, bruises, headaches, upset stomachs, colds and so forth.

Actually, a "leave-health-to-the-doctor" attitude is probably far more of a health threat than self-diagnosis. Important health-building habits—improved diet, exercise, weight control, and avoidance of toxic hazards are a personal responsibility.

And with the gradual clean-up of the patent medicine shelves in drugstores, self-diagnosis is becoming less of a trap for the unwary. Harmful ingredients are being removed from some drugs, and labeling is more truthful. But a lot of work remains to be done, because there are still available drugs which can be abused.

The best course is to take an interest in self-diagnosis and learn to do it right. With a little study and extra care you can avoid many of the pitfalls that trap the compulsive medicine-taker, and you may even learn how to prevent trouble before it happens. Here are some tips:

1. *Learn about your body.* Why be ignorant or self-deceiving about things like the location of your organs, or the value (not harm) of doing some reasonable huff and puff exercise once in a while?

Sure, you learned simple anatomy and physiology in school, but you've probably forgotten more than you care to admit. Pick up a good basic health text from the library or your local paperback store, and give yourself a refresher course.

2. *Start learning about self-help by studying first aid.* Often the doctor can't come when an accident strikes, and you can do plenty to help yourself or others during those important first minutes. Find out how to stop bleeding, prevent shock, and reduce swelling (apply cold packs first).

Books are useful for learning first aid, but by far the best way is to take a course given by the Red Cross or your local **YMCA**.

3. *Think clearly about your problems.* Even if you go to a doctor about an ailment or injury, he's going to have to rely to a large extent on what you tell him about your problem. Think about what you've been doing that might have made you sick, and don't allow yourself to get hooked on pet theories, prejudices, or outlandish ideas.

Medical records are full of stories of people who took powerful drugs for aches and pains when the cause of the trouble was that they were sitting wrong in their chair, sleeping on their arm, or unconsciously leaning against a sharp object for long periods.

A friend of mine wore his belt too tight, and had to get extensive medical tests before it was discovered by his family doctor that the tight belt was the cause of his bellyache. If you think clearly, you can figure such things out for yourself.

4. *Put limits on your self-treatment.* Trying to be independent and self-reliant on health matters is good, but if your problem doesn't go away, see your doctor. That's just common sense, and it's a rule most people follow anyway. But keep in mind that with some problems, prompt medical attention can be important.

5. *Look closely at your own health risks.* Self-diagnosis should mean more than just handling your

own minor illnesses. Far more important is examining your life-style to see if it is increasing your risk of getting sick in the future.

Keep in mind that the really serious health problems of today, such as cancer and heart disease, are caused to a large extent by environmental risks that you expose yourself to voluntarily. And by the time symptoms reveal themselves, it's often too late to cure those diseases.

Your body may not be loaded with chemicals, but if you're not fit you are polluted just as surely as murky air or dirty water are polluted. The heart of a polluted person must work harder to pump blood through all that fat and flab.

Your Heartbeat as a Health Index

A good index of your personal amount of pollution is the rate at which your heart beats. If it chugs along slowly, feel proud. If it clicks a good deal faster than the ticking of a watch, work is needed to get you in shape.

Take your pulse while at rest, say while sitting in your office chair or while relaxing at home. Put two fingertips on the hollow spot in your wrist, or feel the jugular vein in your neck with your whole hand. Don't take your pulse after eating a meal, because your heart is working harder then to supply blood to the stomach for digestion.

Count the number of beats for fifteen seconds, and then multiply by four to get your heart rate per minute. For better accuracy, count beats for thirty seconds.

What is a normal heart rate? Anything from 50 to 100 beats per minute. A pulse in the higher range isn't something to get worked up about, but you'll find that gentle, regular exercise will lower a high pulse and pay big dividends in freeing you from the effects of pollution. Coronary disease is not as common in people with lower pulse rates.

People with regular exercise programs can frequently get their hearts to beat only sixty times a minute, or even slower. Long distance runners sometimes have heart rates of 45 beats a minute. But the best way to test your personal pollution factor is to find out what happens to your heart rate when you do some work.

If you have had a physical recently and know you don't have anything serious wrong with your heart, do this: take your resting pulse and record it on a sheet of paper, then put some old-fashioned dance music on the record player and run in place rhythmically for three minutes.

The three minutes will seem like a long time, but keep at it unless you feel really bushed. At the end of the time, take your pulse again. Then sit down and watch TV or read for five minutes, using a timer of some kind to keep an accurate check of the time. Then take your pulse again and record it. Let another five minutes pass and do the same thing.

Unless your system is badly polluted, your pulse should be back to your normal rate after the 10 minutes. If personal pollution is not your problem, then your pulse will be normal after five minutes.

Some people have the idea that taking your pulse is a sign of being a hypochondriac. They think that only doctors or nurses should be interested in such stuff. That's wrong.

My father, J. I. Rodale, used to be a great pulse-taker. Years ago he realized the importance of ordinary people taking their own pulse, and exercising to get the heart rate lower. Instead of running in place, he would walk hills. He had a book in which

149

he would record his heart-rate daily, sometimes several times daily. After a persistent program of walking up and down hills for several months, he was able to record a very significant drop in his resting heart rate.

Knowing what your heart is doing can be most interesting, and useful. Every heart has a maximum rate above which it isn't safe to go. As you get older and things stiffen up inside, that maximum rate gets lower. Being in my early forties, I know that my cruising speed under stress is about 150 beats a minute. Doing extreme work it can go higher, but that's sort of like driving a car over 100 miles an hour. You might blow something.

Recently, I was out hiking with a pack. It was early evening, about six o'clock, and I had one more steep hill to climb before reaching my campsite for the night. Being hungry, I pushed a little hard and really huffed and puffed. "Take your pulse," something said to me and I did. It was going at 160 beats a minute. So I slowed my climbing a tiny bit and dropped it to 150. Just like a speedometer, the pulse is.

Bowel-Health—A Vital Indicator

Another important indication of health is the efficiency of your bowels. Many people are squeamish when it comes to talking about the bowels, bowel movements, and human wastes in general. That attitude is entirely natural. I am taking the risk of offending your sensitivities to point out the extreme importance of understanding the bowels in making any effort to improve and maintain health. Solid human wastes have an important story to tell. Medical science has used those wastes for many years to

150

diagnose certain infectious and parasitic diseases. The nature of the stool is also an important indicator of a variety of other problems, ranging from spastic colon to celiac disease.

Some facts which have recently come to light indicate that the nature and character of the stool also has a great influence on the origins of some of the most troubling diseases of our age. Diseases which are crippling and fatal, and which are increasing in frequency, are relatively rare among peoples who have a pattern of bowel movements different from Americans. (These people also eat a different type of food, which is part of the story.)

These discoveries about the function of the bowels in preventing serious disease will probably be widely understood one day. However, I doubt that this step ahead in prevention is going to happen by way of traditional medical channels. For one thing, there is a great resistance by the food industry, at the moment, toward promoting the kinds of foods that will lead to bowel health. These products are too cheap to provide a sufficient profit margin. Another reason is that most doctors don't have the training, orientation or persuasive power to teach their patients how to use this new system of prevention.

So I am going to tell you this story and will explain to you certain principles of prevention probably well before (if ever) these ideas become household concepts. And I am going to risk being accused of acting in poor taste by urging you to share this information with your relatives, friends, and even with people you don't know well, but would like to help.

Before getting into the main part of this story I want to explain to you some of the basic biology of solid human wastes. Everyone gives human wastes as short shrift as possible because of the offensive smell with which they have been endowed by nature,

151

for the express purpose of insuring that people stay as far away as possible from fresh, undecomposed fecal matter.

Actually, human wastes and also animal wastes are extremely rich in essential nutrients, and are an important part in the cycle of life which maintains this world as a continually livable place. Nitrogen and both major and minor nutrients of many types are abundant in human wastes. If they are not returned to the land from which those nutrients came, there will be a gradual decline in soil fertility. China has maintained the fertility of its agricultural soils for over four thousand years because human wastes are actually treasured for their properties, and are continually returned to the land.

Furthermore, if human wastes are mixed with ample amounts of cellulose, and are allowed exposure to proper amounts of air and moisture, they are quickly converted by microorganisms into non-smelling, harmless and useful fertilizer. Only when human wastes are allowed to accumulate in isolation in a privy or septic tank do they retain their offensive character for a considerable length of time. Even if human wastes are applied to the soil raw, all disease-causing organisms that they carry are rendered harmless within six months. I certainly don't recommend putting raw wastes on the soil, neverthless it is comforting to know that in half a year, or even less if conditions are favorable, they will be rendered harmless.

The reluctance of people to put wastes on the soil, even after composting, is hard to understand when you realize that millions of gallons of raw sewage are routinely poured into rivers, lakes and oceans each day. And much of that water is then processed for drinking purposes.

Having thus tried to open your eyes to the obvious fact that human wastes are not all bad if handled properly, I will now try to convince you to produce more of them. Yes, that, in a nutshell, is the problem that people in most industrialized countries have with their waste products. Because of the kinds of food they eat, affluent people produce a relatively small amount of solid wastes, and what they do produce lingers much longer in their intestinal tract than what might be considered normal and healthful. And since all human wastes contain substances which are toxic to the intestinal wall, eating foods which linger in the gut increases the chance of harm.

Among rural Africans, colon disease is almost unknown, Burkitt discovered. Yet in America and other western nations colon cancer accounts for twelve to fourteen percent of all cancers. The cause, says Dr. Denis Burkitt, is the kinds of foods that are eaten. Africans eat large amounts of unrefined cereals, and very little sugar or other processed foods. Westerners, on the other hand, eat a highly-refined diet that gives the gut less work to do, so the passage of food is much slower.

The varying speed at which food travels through the human intestinal tract in different cultures has been verified by simple experiments. Food eaten by the average Englishman takes seventy-seven hours to pass through the gut. Tests on English vegetarians showed that they passed their food in forty-nine hours. Yet the average "gastrointestinal transit time" for a rural African is a remarkably short thirty-five hours. And it is interesting to note that one British woman who was moving her bowels every day did not pass a marker pellet until a week after she swallowed it. So even though you may be "regular" on a daily basis, you still can be moving food through your insides very slowly.

There is also a big difference between Africans and Westerners, in the weight of the stools. The average for Africans, in Dr. Burkitt's studies, was 470 grams. But the average Englishman, says Dr. Burkitt, gives forth with "a miserable 108 grams" per stool. "The average stool in England is what I would call just a caricature of a stool," he says.

It's also interesting to note that many rural Africans, especially those on a diet of cornmeal and beans, produce such a large weight of stool that they move their bowels twice a day. In fact, they become quite concerned if they don't have a second bowel movement each day.

To me it appears that all this information about differences in bowel habits between primitive people and residents of industrialized societies should have an enormous impact on the way we live, and, eventually, on our health. If the facts as I have presented them are true—and I am convinced that they are—then simple diet modifications can help insure better health for millions of people in the future, and can reduce the magnitude of the disease crisis that is growing every year.

Why Don't We Change Our Bad Eating Habits?

Unfortunately, there are a number of reasons why people will find changing their diet difficult. Habit is an important factor, especially eating habits. People who are accustomed to eating doughnuts and white bread will find it hard to shake those habits, because no matter what kinds of food you eat you get to like the taste after a while. Furthermore, consumers have formed brand loyalties which they won't want to give up. The food industry has important investments in processing equipment. Also, refined foods have a much longer shelf life than natural foods, an important factor in the supermarket system of food distribution.

The position of the medical establishment on the problem of nutrition needs to be considered. Doctors have not been trained to understand the role of good food in maintaining health, and consequently many have a skeptical attitude.

Dr. Burkitt has been criticized for coming up with a simple answer to cancer, which everyone knows is a very complicated problem. His answer is interesting: "Why should a complicated thing be more likely to be right than a simple thing? All I can say is that we've never yet found a community living on a high-residue diet that didn't have a minimal incidence of bowel cancer. We've never yet found a people who have gone from a high to low-residue diet who haven't subsequently developed the non-infective diseases of the bowel."

So even though the general public's awakening to the value of more natural foods to bowel health is likely to be slow, there's no reason why you can't use that information now. And there's even less reason why you should hesitate to pass this information along to others.

Using Dr. Burkitt's ideas is not really a complicated task. The easiest thing for me to do to explain his technique of diet modification would be to draw up a list of "don't" foods—things that you shouldn't eat. But I think that it's far better to focus attention on the positive, on the things that you and your friends and relatives *should* eat to get your food moving faster through your intestines, and provide insurance against bowel disease.

Dr. Burkitt puts great emphasis on bran, the outer part of the wheat that is removed during milling. In his household, an eight-gram spoonful of bran is added to each person's food every day. (Bran can be purchased in many health food stores, and perhaps even in special health food departments in supermarkets.) The Burkitts also eat real whole grain bread, the kind that they make themselves from whole wheat flour. It's important to realize that much of the sliced, plastic-wrapped bread that is labeled as whole wheat is, in fact, not. It has some whole grain flour in it, usually, but is dyed dark with caramel to give it a brown color. That kind of bread will be of little or no use for the purposes we are recommending.

Eating bran regularly may take some getting used to. The taste is not offensive, but your innards could well take a few weeks to adjust to the extra work. That is perfectly normal and will pass in a short time. And while you're starting on the bran regime, start cutting down on your sugar intake, because sugar is one of the refined foods that has a detrimental effect on the gut, in Dr. Burkitt's opinion.

My own belief is that corn meal is an important food to include in your diet, for bowel health. Rural Africans eat a good deal of corn meal mush and other foods made from unrefined corn. That has been pointed out by Dr. Burkitt and by others working on the same problem.

I have found that the most convenient and the tastiest way to eat corn regularly is in the form of homemade corn pones. In fact, I have been eating them for years because I like the taste much better than the taste of bread, and I value them even more now that I know of their bowel-bulking action. Here is the recipe:

Heat several cups of water to boiling. While it is heating, put three cups of *white* corn meal and a half-teaspoon of salt in a mixing bowl. If you can get raw peanut flour, add about one-half cup of that, and you can also add some sesame seeds and/or caraway seeds.

Slowly pour the boiling water and one-third cup of corn oil into the meal at the same time. Stir thoroughly. Use only enough of the water to make a firm dough, not too wet.

After the mixture cools, form into about 15 cakes with your hands. I let the imprints of my fingers remain to save time. Bake on a greased pan for 35 to 40 minutes in a 375 degree oven. They are done when the edges get well-browned.

There is more to good diet than vitamins, minerals, fats, carbohydrates and other essential nutrients. We must eat to provide the proper physical environment in the gut, if we are to avoid many painful and expensive diseases of civilization.

They Don't Feel Sick—but They Don't Feel Great Either

But what we eat isn't the only thing that counts in the way we feel. Many people tell me they don't really feel sick, but they don't feel great either. They say they have no pep, no ambition. Is there *really* a way to gain more energy? Yes, there certainly is, and it's a completely natural way.

In most cases lack of energy has its roots in our machine-age culture. Muscles that are seldom used get weak and lose power. Our human "energy crisis" is usually as simple as that. If you have the kind of weakness and lassitude that seems pathological, see your doctor. Tiredness throughout the day can be a symptom of illness.

Scientific studies pinpoint lack of fitness as the prime cause of fatigue. Evalyn S. Gendel, M.D., of

157

the Kansas State Department of Health recently studied sixty-seven young women who she said were typical examples of "the tired, complaining, cross female." Many reported fatigue and a general tired feeling.

All the women were examined medically, and also given physical fitness tests. None of the complainers were actually sick, said Dr. Gendel. But those who complained the loudest about being tired tended to score low on the physical fitness tests. If you lack energy, lack of fitness could be your problem.

Of course, exercise is the remedy. Yet exercise—if approached directly—requires a degree of motivation and willpower that most people can't muster. They start a program of calisthenics or jogging, then drop out when the weather turns bad or their muscles ache.

Enthusiasm is the real answer to the problem of feeling better and gaining energy, says Eric Taylor, author of *Fitness After 40* and a former chief fitness instructor for the Royal Air Force. "Your mind governs the way you feel," he says, "and the vigor of your emotions can revitalize your muscles." But you do have to look after your body sensibly, he says, with rest, exercise, and the right food. Eric Taylor cites evidence that enthusiasm and excitement stimulate the adrenal glands to pump hormones into the bloodstream, which help the liver to release energy fuel.

Some medical authorities also give mental attitudes credit for vigor. Drs. Peter J. Steinchron and David J. LaFia say that "Cheerfulness, courage, optimism, faith and equanimity produce chemical changes in your body that promote health." Those attitudes stimulate the endocrine glands, say the two doctors.

How can you put your own emotions to work helping you to feel better, and to gain energy?

Get excited about your potential for feeling better. Excitement turns on your personal chemistry of physical strength. Make a list of the things you would like to do if you felt that you had the strength and drive. Think of the fun you can have when you start drawing on new stores of energy.

Build a good foundation for your energy-building campaign. Start doing the things that everyone knows are important to health, like getting enough sleep, eating moderately, drinking less. Always keep in mind your ultimate goal of building more energy and feeling better. That will give you the motivation to take a new interest in sensible health habits.

Start exercising, but be gradual and gentle. Decide in advance that building energy is going to be a long-term project. Walk, don't run, toward your goal. Walking, as a matter of fact, is one of the best forms of exercise, and a wonderful energy builder.

Find ways to measure your growing energy potential. See how long you can walk now before getting tired. Stress yourself slightly, perhaps by walking two or three hours at a stretch. Every few weeks, give yourself the same walking test and check for energy improvement. Get yourself a good pair of of hiking shoes to prevent sore feet.

Try gentle exercise as a remedy for end-of-the day slump. Move around in the evening. Go out for a breath of fresh air, swing your arms, jog in place. Do anything except admit that tiredness is inevitable. It isn't. Frequently, only a little movement will lift your emotions and get your glands pumping energy fuel into your system.

Vitamins Are Essential

What vitamins should I take? That is the most common question I am asked. Unfortunately, there is no easy answer. Nobody knows exactly what amount of each vitamin or mineral is needed by each individual person. The metabolism and dietary requirements of people vary. Even exhaustive tests given by a nutrition researcher might fail to reveal the exact amount of vitamins and minerals that will benefit you.

The National Research Council does publish recommended dietary allowances, but they are frankly stated to be guides for use in mass feeding in institutions, not directly applicable to individual needs. And those allowances are on the low side, because they are taken primarily to prevent deficiency diseases, like scurvy and pellagra. The newer idea that good nutrition can increase human efficiency has not been given sufficient attention.

Different people live different kinds of lives. If you have a large garden of your own and are able to get much of your food in natural and fresh form, you probably need fewer food supplements. Do you smoke and thereby use up some of your vitamin C intake? Do you live in a polluted area? Do you do heavy, manual work, requiring extra calories? All those factors influence your need for food supplements.

So the first step in answering the question "What vitamins should I take?" is to understand that your needs are largely individualized and personal. You are going to have to decide for yourself what vitamins to take, adjusting your intake as you gain more information about yourself and your environment.

Many people solve the vitamin-decision problem by taking an all-in-one type of tablet. These are perfectly acceptable, especially as insurance against routine deficiencies. But the separate tablets and capsules offer more flexibility, allowing you to increase or decrease each nutrient in your program based on your own ideas of what you need. That's what I do.

A New Tomorrow

What is to become of the human race? I am an optimist. My vision of our future is a hopeful one. We are going to survive as a nation and as individuals. But there will be changes in the way we live as we approach the bottom of the world's barrel of resources, particularly oils and minerals. The famous "American way of life," which most of us have become accustomed to, is going to change drastically.

Many smart people have seen what is happening (some have seen the day of resource reckoning coming for 30 years or more) and have been working on survival programs. They have been trying to build a way of life that is insulated as much as possible from shortsighted living, in which "success" goes mainly to those people who know how to use up resources the quickest. Their goal is to try instead to live their lives in a posture that will allow them to remain standing, when the rest of society begins to crumple under the burden of being champion consumers, in a day when there isn't much left to consume.

The most outstanding example of people who have learned to stand on their own two feet are the members of the rural religious sects, who have woven prescriptions against technological change into their faith itself. They are the Amish, the Hutterites, and some branches of the Mennonite Church. Shortages of electricity bother them little, since they still illuminate their homes with kerosene lamps or Coleman lanterns, and don't use air-conditioning or electric cookstoves either. Rationing of food wouldn't hit them at all, since they grow more than they need. In all areas, their consumption of mineral and energy resources is but a fraction of that of the average family.

True, their lives are more primitive than ours, their homes less comfortable, and their children not educated to fill leadership roles in industry, education and government. But in a sense these fundamentalist religious farmers have a much greater freedom than the average person. It is a freedom from slavery to possessions, to status, and to the world-wide balance of trade. And that freedom goes a long way toward compensating these hard-working people for their sacrifices of personal comfort.

Many efforts have been made to duplicate the kind of land-oriented independence that the Amish and other sects enjoy, but they have not succeeded totally. That is because religious faith of a unique kind is indispensible to what they are doing. Their faith calls on them to help each other in time of need —to gather together to build barns, to plow the fields of sick brethren, and to sell each other land at less-than-market prices. They substitute cooperation for the competition that rules our world, and build mutual strength. It is a great and successful formula, but can't be imitated without the glue of a unique religious tradition.

How To Stand on Your Own Two Feet

So if we are going to stand on our own two feet, we will probably have to do it either alone, or in very small groups. And the best way for us to do that is by what has come to be called homesteading. I don't mean homesteading on the frontier pattern— the building of a farm from scratch on 160 acres of free government land. Those days are gone, probably forever. The modern homesteader is usually a part-time farmer or large-scale gardener who creates a large part of the food, recreation, and possibly even fuel and clothing from a piece of land that is operated somewhat like a subsistence farm. Most modern homesteaders work full time in offices or factories, or are retired. They have some other source of income, because it is almost impossible these days to live entirely on the fruits of labor on the land. A homestead is great for producing food, but there are other bills to pay too.

Even homesteading is beyond the means, and possibly the desires, of the great majority of people. There are limits of land, of time, and of money that place the total organic homestead just too far from the grasp of all but a minority—at least for the present. But that problem doesn't lessen the need for independence created by the growing shortage of resources. Nor does it dilute the feeling of a growing number of people that now is the time to learn to stand on your own feet.

So we are going to have to compromise, to bring some of the elements of homesteading into our lives. In that way, while we won't be able to achieve total protection from resource-crunch catastrophe, we can at least maneuver into a position that will enable us to ride out the storm more easily.

First, we must shift gears psychologically. It's important to face up to the idea of making do with less, of getting by without all the expensive material things and services we're so accustomed to. Accept it as a challenge.

We must grow more of our own food. If you

have access to any land at all—your own, a community garden plot, or even a rootftop garden or window box—put it to work producing food. Do it organically right from the start, because costly chemical fertilizers and poison sprays are going to be too expensive anyway when the energy and resource crisis really sets in.

All of us should try to can and store more food. By learning how to process your own food and keep it through the winter, you'll be avoiding one of the biggest added expenses in your present food bill. Arrange for a cool, dry place where you can store root crops like carrots, potatoes, turnips and beets, as well as dry, natural foods like beans and grains in bulk.

We can make it a practice to buy more simple, natural foods that keep well and supply good nutrition. Stock up on dried beans, which can be sprouted later for extra vitamins and food value.

"For everyone, even for us who live in bounteous America, the time will probably come when food and other necessities are unobtainable," says Esther Dickery in her book, *Passport to Survival* (Bookcraft Publishers). "Our urban society is particularly vulnerable.

She recommends we all stock up on basic "survival foods." Wheat, powdered milk and honey top her list, as well as peanut butter, tomato juice, soybeans, dried green peas, lentils, millet, corn, dried fruit, raisins and nuts. Wheat and soybeans can always be sprouted for variety and extra food value.

Give more thought to the economy of food supplements. They're usually much cheaper sources of vitamins and minerals than the "protective" foods—fish, fruits, nuts and vegetables, to name a few. If you find that you can't get enough of the foods you know you need to stay healthy, be sure that your food supplement program is adequate to cover your needs.

Buy some land. If you aren't already a land-owner, now is the time. Demand will soon send the price of dwindling land parcels out of sight for the average homesteader. And without land, you're going to have trouble raising the kind of harvests you'll need to feed your family.

Get tools. Learn to take care of simple repairs around the house. Develop some home skill or craft to be ready for the advent of home industry. When harder times come, we'll all be looking for secondary income sources. You might even consider growing earthworms for gardeners, or for fish bait. Beekeep-ing or raising specialty crops such as berries or herbs are other income possibilities.

Get to know your neighbors better. Learn to share equipment and special skills. Become familiar with the way food-buying co-ops work. We may all have to work together someday to get by.

We must resolve to use less energy. Buy a smaller car with fewer cylinders and less of an appe-tite for gasoline. Get a bicycle for shorter trips and everyday errands. When power brownouts come, a kerosene lamp or two will surely come in handy. And when the energy pinch really sets in, air condi-tioning is going to be one of the first things to go. Start cutting back now on cooling *and* heating. Re-discover the natural rhythm of the four seasons.

Build up your health through good diet and adequate exercise. Become more health-conscious in general so that you'll be better able to withstand the stress of shortages and harder times. After all, doctor bills are a burden even in the best of times.

Above all, don't be discouraged. In our society where overconsumption is the rule, cutting back a little on energy and other resource use would still leave us with an enviable standard of living. If *all* of us are willing to make some small changes in the way we live, our future will remain bright. We will survive, as a nation and as individuals.

Tomorrow's Health Trends 10

Everything changes rapidly these days, and food tastes are no exception. New kinds of food pop onto supermarket shelves with increasing regularity. Old-favorite foods pass out of style almost as if they were last year's brand of auto or washing machine.

Beef has become the prestige food of our affluent society. Since 1952, consumption has jumped from 62 pounds per person a year to 116 pounds. Popularity of chicken zoomed from 20 pounds per person a year in 1952 to 43 pounds in 1973.

Convenience food consumption has also gone up, but not quite as dramatically. Frozen, canned and packaged foods of all kinds gain steadily in popularity, while use of fresh fruits and vegetables declines. Grain products, especially bread, have been in a long-time slump as people turn their attention to more glamorous foods.

Why do these shifts occur? Are they caused by a change in what people perceive to be good taste in food, or are there other reasons? Can rising incomes alone explain what is happening?

My opinion is that the most significant changes in food preferences aren't initiated in the kitchen or dining room, but are imposed on people by marketing goals of large food companies and restaurant chains. Simply stated, some foods are more profitable to sell than others and, not surprisingly, those foods gradually become more popular.

Consider the lowly potato, for example. In its fresh form it holds little glamour for the cook. There is also not much money to be made selling fresh potatoes.

If a spud is transformed into a frozen French fry, however, it becomes America's second most profitable food item. Only soft drinks offer greater mark-up possibilities. So it is not surprising to note that frozen French fried potatoes have enjoyed a spectacular 460 percent increase in popularity since 1960. Consumption of fresh potatoes is way off in the same period.

The same thing has happened to other vegetables and fruits. In fresh form, produce spoils easily. So the public finds itself not liking fresh vegetables and fruits as much. Sales of frozen and canned vegetables are up, and so are sales of canned fruit juice.

Fast food outlets and vending machines are also exerting their powerful muscle on American eating habits. Only foods that don't spoil easily and offer significant profits lend themselves to mass merchandising by such outlets. We end up gradually changing our food preferences to fit in with the trend.

Even the breakfast meal is vulnerable to profit motives. High-profit baked goods and packaged cereals are holding their own, while egg consumption levels are going down.

Sugar, the leading "empty calorie" food, stays at the level of more than 100 pounds per person each year. Clearly, diet shifts have not been in the direction of more healthful eating, at least in the area of sweeteners.

Rising Prices and the Trend toward Diet Change

Unfortunately, rising prices for food commodities are likely to accelerate the trend toward diet change. Not only is the family budget under pressure, but food processors also find themselves faced with higher bills for raw materials, plus other increased costs of doing business. Their response will be to try to sell more of the processed foods, so that they can enjoy the markup that goes to those who alter food in some way.

What is the best way out of the problem of food future shock for people who have to watch pennies? Self-discipline is crucial, limiting your food selections to more natural foods which offer high nutritional value at lower prices, but which may take more time to prepare.

Home gardening is a good alternative for those people who have land available—even if it's only a small plot. Millions are now finding that a backyard plot can produce hundreds of dollars worth of excellent food each season.

The kind of food gardeners grow at home is becoming more difficult to find in commercial markets, even at the peak of the season. Though *you* can grow high-quality produce at home, there's not enough profit in good fresh vegetables to keep the wheels of the food distribution mechanism for commercial markets turning rapidly.

The situation promises to get worse. What is the answer? One thing we can do is become health minded.

Health "Nuts" Are Healthier

Continual attacks on health foods, organic foods and even vitamins have tended to conceal one unarguable fact—health-minded people are healthier than other people. They eat better food, get more exercise, depend less on doctors and drugs, and even have a happier outlook on life.

Strange as it seems there are few formal, controlled studies that probe the effect of food faddism and unorthodox health interests on personal health levels. Universities and government agencies have shown almost no interest in investigating the health of "health nuts," and the food industry hasn't tackled the subject yet either.

Health superiority of people who eat natural foods is clear, however, and is easily revealed by informal surveys. John Glyer, a third-year medical student at California Medical College in San Francisco, recently published the results of a series of interviews he had with people who believe in what he calls "diet healing." They were largely patrons of youth-oriented, natural food stores and also traditional health food stores.

Health food store customers, according to Glyer, "have effectively eliminated such bad habits as drinking, smoking, overeating, and chemical control of their bodies through 'uppers' and 'downers.' "

The ranks of "health nuts" are also replete with examples of personal achievement at advanced age—further evidence that paying attention to personal health pays dividends in vitality. Elmer Onstott of Ferguson, Missouri, for example, walked the Appalachian Trail at the age of 69, eating only seeds, nuts and raw vegetables. And Larry Lewis, who still works as a banquet waiter at the age of 100-plus jogs every day and watches his diet carefully.

Many establishment nutritionists and health experts are unimpressed. There is almost total lack of sympathy with the movement at high academic levels, although everyone agrees that the health food idea is here to stay.

Antagonism toward the Health Food Movement

Why has this antagonism developed? Why are efforts of ordinary people to help themselves to health scorned instead of supported? There are several reasons:

Commercial exploitation. The business side of the health food field turns off many outside observers. They claim that some health foods are no better than supermarket foods, and cost more. That's sometimes true, yet it's also true that health food stores sell, at reasonable prices, many good products which aren't available in supermarkets.

Strangeness. Enthusiasm for good health sends out odd vibrations to someone tuned to a totally scientific view of life. Yoga, metaphysics and other forms of spirituality are part of the food scene to so-called faddists, and they help to create a meaningful and pleasant routine of life for them. Yet that kind of thinking is foreign to most nutritionists, who can't see why food should amount to more than nourishment and flavor.

Other wars. Fights over fluoridation, mass inoculation programs and other traditional public health measures have made long-term enemies. Establishment health scientists don't see how they can talk on the same level with people who fight programs they consider essential.

171

Health conscious people, on the other hand, see their regimens as a kind of rebellion against dangerous stupidity.

Freedom to die happy. Although many doctors are now urging their patients to eat and exercise more wisely, most medical men tend to feel that dissipation is one of life's pleasures. They hesitate to advise the kind of strict diet routine that health enthusiasts follow willingly.

I don't believe this antagonism toward the health food movement will continue in all areas. There are many indications that "times are changing."

At last the schools are becoming aware of the importance of good nutrition. Classes in healthful eating are becoming of major interest to schools and colleges catering to students of all ages. Often these courses combine nutrition education of the formal, technical kind with such closely-related subjects as gardening and physical fitness.

The future looks even brighter. I predict that food, nutrition and the whole idea of living naturally and organically are soon going to become as basic as reading, writing and arithmetic in the curricula of schools. And people of all ages will sign up to take courses that will, once and for all, explain the mysteries of vitamins, minerals, enzymes, and nutrients of all kinds.

The beginning of the boom in nutrition studies —that we are seeing now—is a coming forth from The Dark Ages. Until recently, nutrition has been a suppressed subject, not only ignored but actually held down. As a result, the average person in this country simply does not understand how to select a diet that will keep weight down, improve fitness and well-being, and assure health into the retirement years.

But we can see ahead to a time when people know enough about food to select a truly beneficial diet. I am sure that there will soon be a nutritionally-educated segment of the population that will be a powerful force for improvement of food offered for sale, because they will select what is good based on a true understanding of nutritional principles.

How Americans Arrived at Their Nutritional Ignorance

To understand why Americans are about to escape from nutrition ignorance, you should know how we got there in the first place.

For many years politics and national pride fed the shallow concept that "America is the best-fed nation on earth." The trappings of affluence and bulging supermarkets were confused with true nutritional adequacy. People were overfed but undernourished, and only the so-called food faddists realized that.

Nutrition teachers were for a long time the captives of the food industry. Unfortunately many still are, but the number of independent teachers is growing rapidly. The big money in food is made by processing and manipulating it, which also usually reduces its nutritional value. Some of those profits were used in subtle ways to capture the loyalties of home economists, nutritionists, and health educators.

Criticism of bad food was brushed off effectively as "faddism." Much of the energy of nutrition teachers was devoted to cracking down on health food "nuts" and "quacks," distracting the public's attention from the instructors' own brand of false teaching.

Poor education wasn't the only reason why national eating habits sank so low. Pockets of poverty

173

caused some people to suffer from borderline starvation. And the sheer technological power of man to manipulate food brought us too far away from natural goodness, without any compensating philosophy of eating that could be understood by the mass of people. Why are those days ending? Because of the ecology movement, mainly. People are waking up to the fact that environmental quality is worsening. First, the air and water claimed their attention. Then they began to realize that there is an ecology of the body as well as of the biosphere. And environmental scientists helped too by looking for—and finding— pollutants in foods. Worries about pesticides, mercury, and depleted nutrients were on everyone's mind.

The teaching of ecology is now almost mandatory in all schools, even kindergartens. What used to be nature study is now environmental education, and what better way to teach people about the environment than to discuss their own personal ecology, using food as an example? By that route, the study of nutrition is being taken from the exclusive hands of the old-line home economists and is being packaged and sold by teachers who are in tune with concerns of the day.

Response to a Need

One of the best of this new breed of teacher is Walter Tulecke, a botanist at the Science Institute of Antioch College in Ohio, an institution long known for innovation and inspired programs. Reacting to a letter to the editor in the school paper three years ago requesting a seminar in nutrition, Professor Tulecke worked out an undergraduate general education course in nutrition. He expected 10 to 15 students to show up, but 120 came to the first meeting.

Breaking out of the traditional bounds of nutrition education, leaving the biases and strictures behind, he planned a course with many innovations. Lectures were given only twice a week. Many outside speakers were brought in. Movies were used, and field trips were held often. Students went to a hospital, a brewery, an organic farm, and held some of their discussion sessions in supermarkets. They learned to prepare a dietary intake chart for a day, weighing all their food and determining its nutritional value.

"One of the unusual aspects of this course is the serving of food in class," Tulecke says. That sounds like it would be routine for the study of the science of food, but you can't imagine how restrictive some concepts of food teaching have been. A clue to the tone of the class is revealed by the listing of foods Walter Tulecke says have been served: homemade cottage cheese, peanut bread, garbanzo patties, high-protein muffins, survival food for backpacking, soybean casserole, kasha, yogurt, and so forth.

There is a garden too. "A quarter of an acre of golf course turf was turned under, fertilized with manure, campus leaves, and compost, and planted to vegetables of many different types," Tulecke says. That organic garden, also worked by townspeople, became a focal point of the nutrition studies.

"The garden," adds Tulecke, "was a good place for discussions and it frequently became a small learning center related to nutrition, soils, biological control and many other subjects."

The most important thing about a class like this—a feeling which is hard to put into words—is the sheer *freedom* of learning a subject like nutrition when it is taught in the new atmosphere of openness. Released from the need to follow the party line of the food processors, a teacher of nutrition can make the subject exciting. Under the old system, nutrition teachers were afraid to get their students too excited about the subject for fear the youngsters would turn into faddists. That's true! Caring too much about food, becoming passionate about its health values, is a sign of pathology to a traditional nutritionist.

The new wave rolls on, though, over the heads of the old-timers. Walter Tulecke is just one of the new breed. Even more radical, yet with perhaps even more pertinent academic orientation, is Mrs. Norma Westcott, an innovative and dedicated health teacher working for the state of New York. Her new type of health and nutrition program is called "Prescription for Life," and her students are 310 eighth graders of the Shendehowa Central School District near Albany.

They've Given Up on Adults

"Public Health experts have just about given up on the current generation of adults," the *New York Times* says in reporting on Westcott's work. One of her goals is to train young people to be general health counselors—to teach preventive medicine concepts to their friends and even to their parents.

In fact, these kids can be pretty hard on their parents. "My mother is killing me," one student reported to his class. How? By making him eat a breakfast with too much fat.

Westcott's students learn more than nutrition. They know how to take each other's pulse, blood pressure, and can even work electrocardiogram machines. After exercising regularly, they see how their hearts become trained, and how their bodies can do more work with less strain on their cardiovascular systems.

The idea of making eighth graders into health

counselors is fascinating, to say the least. It is a practical idea too, and a great example of the kind of nutritional and health-education advances that can be made once people start looking beyond the facade of prestige and degrees that has entangled the health-care professions. Many people are now thinking along that route, not just Westcott. New ways must be found to teach people rapidly to help others to better health.

If you want to get on the bandwagon:

Check your local elementary and secondary schools to see if they are teaching nutrition in an environmentally-oriented way. Call the school superintendent and ask him. If they're not yet doing it, write a letter suggesting that they get started. Offer your help.

See what courses are now available that you can take yourself. Look for nutrition and human ecology on the adult education programs of local colleges, especially community colleges. If they aren't yet available, suggest that they be started.

Get more serious about your non-classroom nutrition and health education. Do more reading in natural science. Check your local library for semi-technical books on nutrition and health and invest time in studying them. The purpose of that effort is to prepare for the time, which I'm sure is coming soon, when the definition of a nutritionist or of a health educator is going to be expanded tremendously.

A Plan for Health Consultation by Mail

There is no question that a great need exists for education of adults about health matters. Many people are needlessly falling victim to chronic, degenerative diseases because they do not have the knowledge and motivation to select a proper diet, avoid toxic hazards, attain an adequate level of physical fitness, and avoid needless physical stress.

Traditional methods of public health education have produced extremely disappointing results. In fact, it is generally agreed that the failure to be able to quantify any tangible results from almost all formal adult health education efforts is a cause of the stagnation that exists in this field.

There are several reasons why health education is a difficult challenge. There is no need to list those reasons here, as they are well known. However, I would like to point out two facts.

First, a market for health information exists, as evidenced by the remarkable growth and continued expansion of the popular health movement. The reason for that growth is that the popular health movement treats health in a positive sense—as a talent that can be developed through study, practice and effort.

People are teaching themselves to adjust their living habits so that they can prevent disease and lead healthier lives. There is no longer any doubt about the role that fitness and lifelong healthful living habits play in our well-being. Degenerative illnesses have now been documented as "diseases of civilization" in study after study. Not all such diseases are in that category, of course, but heart disease and cancer have been found to be associated quite closely with environmental hazards in our "advanced" society. Many of those hazards are avoidable, but only if people know what the hazards are, and have the will to avoid them. The people in the new health movement are learning and teaching the kind of health concepts desperately needed today if we are to avoid the problems fostered by the currently accepted dietary regimens and sedentary life styles.

The popular health movement also equates health with personal efficiency and lifelong satisfaction, not merely with the absence of disease. There are no "outer limits" to health when it is looked at in a positive way.

Physicians are so closely associated with the word health, in the minds and imaginations of people, that a vacuum in health teaching and consulting has been created. This is due to a fear that the preserve of doctors might be infringed on by someone not trained by the present health establishment, but someone who ventures to tell others what they should do to try to make their lives more healthful. If that vacuum is not filled with health information, it will be filled with disease, slowly but inevitably. That is happening now, and it's time we turn things around.

The second consideration is that health education needs vary from one person to another. Almost all existing health education programs are general and non-individualized in nature. There is almost no way for the great majority of consumers to get individualized advice and consultation in a coordinated way about all phases of health education. Personalized health education, were it available on a large scale, would likely produce measurable results. Motivation to follow health-building recommendations would be increased by an individualized program.

The present methods of consumer health education also fall short. President Nixon, in his health message to the 92nd Congress, made the same point. "We have given remarkably little attention to the health education of our people. Most of our current efforts in this area are fragmented and haphazard. A public advertisement once a week, a newspaper ar-

179

ticle once another week, a short lecture now and then. There is no national instrument, no central force, to stimulate and coordinate a comprehensive health education program," he emphasized.

It is because of this general lack of health knowledge that millions of our young people have decided the pleasures of narcotics outweigh their health hazards, and millions of the rest of us have decided that obesity is preferable to giving up favorite foods, and that a weak heart, weak legs and a paunchy stomach can be better tolerated than the possible inconvenience and hard work of vigorous physical exercise.

I believe one solution to this problem is to train health workers who could serve as personal consultants. These consulting health educators would receive training in diet and nutrition, physical fitness, environmental improvement, counseling and motivational techniques.

Progress toward creating a profession of consulting health educators has been slow, even though evidence of a need for that service accumulates at ever-more-rapid rates. A big problem is the interdisciplinary nature of personalized health education. There are utopian overtones to the suggestion that one person could be trained (at least in the near future) to provide authoritative counseling on a broad spectrum of matters related to health. The schools of public health and health education which are now in a severe financial bind, do not have the resources available to experiment with a training program that might not show results for several years.

Instead I propose that similar personal health consultation could be carried out through the mail by a team of advisors—people drawn from the ranks of existing professions. Here is a theoretical description of the operation of an individualized health-education-by-mail program:

Information about the service would be made known to the public through publicity of various types, including word-of-mouth, referrals from doctors, YM/WCA's, Jewish Community Centers, releases to newspapers, mail ads, and so forth.

At the outset applicants would receive a complete description of the service, including an agreement saying what the service would provide, and detailing its limits. It would be made clear that in no way does this service offer help with the diagnosis or treatment of any disease or condition. It would provide advice only (and motivation to follow that advice), aimed at helping the client to maintain health in the future.

After completing the application, clients would receive a packet of forms and questionnaires designed to elicit information the panel would use as the basis for its initial advice. Some of the information areas to be covered could include:

1. A physical description of the client and his environment—including height, weight, birth date, age, sex, occupation, type of residence, family environment, activity pattern, history of smoking—and those portions of the client's medical history that would be necessary to anyone attempting to give effective and safe health advice. In certain instances, doctors' recommendations would be included.

2. Another form would provide the client with the opportunity to explain intangible factors that could influence his health-preserving program. Those would include his specific health aims, preferences in sport and recreation, tastes in food, and the reasons why he thinks he has failed or succeeded in previous health-improvement efforts.

3. Finally, a group of daily logs would be provided for the client to use in recording, for three or four days, all activities which would have an effect

on the design of a specific health-improvement plan for him. Primarily, that would mean recording the type and amount of all foods eaten, exercise taken, and exposure to specific health risks, such as pollution.

These completed forms would be returned by mail to a panel of health advisors. All the members of the panel would be trained and licensed health educators, nutritionists, home economists, physical educators, and environmental experts. In my opinion it would also be necessary for experts on motivational techniques and communications to contribute input to the panel, either as advisors or auxiliary technicians.

After the Forms Are Evaluated . . .

After the completed forms had been evaluated, the clients would receive responses pointing out the health threats to which they are most likely exposing themselves, and advising techniques to use in creating a more healthful personal environment.

Referrals could be made to specific health improvement programs available in the client's locality, such as group exercise programs, anti-smoking clinics, etc. But the primary emphasis would be on supplying written information that would help to inform and motivate the client. Some of that information could be supplied in originally-typed form, and other parts as standard printed material. In the initial stages some reward system would be devised to encourage the client to continue to follow healthy habits.

Most important of all would be the continuity of the program. A dialogue would be maintained with the client through the mail and frequent reminders about the need to follow programs started would be sent. As much as possible, the mail dialogue would represent a genuine and original exchange of ideas between the client and the panel, or a designated member of the panel.

After pre-determined periods of time, new physical description forms would be submitted to the client to measure the effectiveness of the program. Other reporting means could also be devised.

This description of a mail health consultation-program is theoretical, so it obviously is open to change and expansion when implemented. Clients would be asked to pay for this service, at the outset, but development funding would be needed to carry start-up costs and overhead. First a pilot program should be created, whose purpose would be to test and adapt the program for later use on a larger scale. This pilot project should be operated by a non-profit organization.

The main reasons I recommend development of a personalized health education program through the mail are as follows, not necessarily in order of importance.

1. Economy.
2. Saving time. The consultant's time is not used to gather information, but only to respond.
3. Practicality. There is less need to train one person in all facets of health education. Different parts of the advice program can be supplied by different members of the team of advisors.
4. Insulation against efforts by clients to get diagnosis or treatment of problems that require the care of a physician. It is easier to cut off such requests by mail than in person.

I believe that this program could be very effective. True, health education has been the most disappointing of fields, but so little effort has been made to personalize health education, and as far as I know there is almost no way that the average person can get personal answers to comprehensive questions about health today. There are fitness advisors, diet advisors, drug abuse counselors, anti-smoking counselors, and so forth, but no one person or group to whom a person can go for a comprehensive program of health maintenance and maximization.

The direct-contact nature of this program also provides a simple way to measure the effectiveness of health education efforts.

Would people use this service? Would the average person be willing to fill in the forms and take the advice? Those questions can only be answered by testing the program. I am sure *some* people would welcome this service and use it enthusiastically and effectively. How many, remains to be determined. By using the mails, they can be reached effectively wherever they live, thereby overcoming problems of geographical location.

Through public education and self-education, we can learn to use our human resources to full advantage. New China has done a good job of this. Their system of medicine is a splendid example.

Let's Adapt the Barefoot Doctor Idea

The barefoot doctor holds the star position in Chinese medicine, in my opinion. These hard-working people have, for the first time in history, brought effective medical care to hundreds of millions of rural Chinese who never before got any kind of professional medical attention at all.

About 80 percent of the Chinese people live in the country, often in villages that have no good road or rail connections to nearby towns. The concentration of people in those isolated areas is mind-boggling by our standards. Regular doctors almost never bothered to go there in the past, because of poverty and the transportation problems.

Now, every hamlet has its barefoot doctor, a person trained to handle the routine, repetitive kind of health problems that don't require the attention of someone with an extensive medical education.

Barefoot doctors are mainly young people—most appear to be under thirty. They have had three to six months training at a hospital or army medical unit in basic prevention techniques, first aid, diagnosis and treatment of roughly 100 common diseases. They go back to school for a week or so every six months, and are checked on weekly by a medical doctor sent around by the commune hospital.

At least half the time, the average barefoot doctor works in the fields, or does other non-medical jobs. But in the early morning and late afternoon and evening, he or she holds office hours in a small office, catering to the health needs of other members of the brigade. Often the barefoot doctor will make house calls in the evening, checking on bedridden patients.

Perhaps the affectionate title of barefoot before the word doctor has helped downgrade these remarkable people in our eyes, and caused their work to be overlooked. Actually they are highly respected, and perhaps even prosperous by Chinese standards. And because they serve the peasants, who have often been helpless in the face of disease, the barefoot doctors are honored.

Of course, these partly-trained doctors do make mistakes, but my impression is that problems are kept to a minimum by two factors. First, fully-trained doctors are always nearby to give help, especially with serious cases. And second, the barefoot doctors work mainly with herbal medicines, often collected right in the brigade's area. These plant drugs seldom cause the side effects commonly experienced with synthetic drugs.

The effectiveness of the million-and-a-quarter barefoot doctors with their herbal medicines was brought home to me when I visited a commune hospital near Canton recently. Although the hospital had 33 beds and 12 doctors, it had very few bed patients. The 60,000 residents of the commune were also being served by almost 30 barefoot doctors and an equal number of midwives, out in the production brigades. Their work, and their drugs, must have been producing results. The light patient load of the hospital was evidence of that.

Do we need barefoot doctors here in the U.S.? Probably we could use a few in isolated areas, where regular doctors are simply not available. But I'm convinced that we have a big need for a similar large body of young people working in a slightly different field—health education.

The main threat to life here is not uncared-for acute disease, but the slow, debilitating effect of overeating, underexercising, smoking, drinking, drug abuse and similar self-inflicted hazards. Regular doctors don't have the time, and often not even the training, to counter these problems.

Health educators, trained quickly to be able to advise people how best to build a more healthful style of life, could have a quick and positive effect on national well-being. They wouldn't have to know about disease and diagnosis techniques at all, and wouldn't function as junior doctors. But they could learn to tell people how to eat right, exercise safely, and motivate themselves to follow health-building routines permanently.

A closer look at China's successful barefoot doctor experience might convince even the skeptics that —with the proper help and advice—people can learn to help themselves to better health.

Anesthetized with Needles, Not Chemicals

Another highlight of my trip to China in 1973 was the opportunity to watch an abdominal operation done on a patient who was anesthetized only with needles, not with chemicals as is the exclusive custom in the United States. That chance came during my visit to Shanghai—specifically at the Hsinhua (New China) Hospital.

There is a tendency to call this kind of anesthesia "acupuncture," which is not completely accurate. Acupuncture is a technique of Chinese traditional medicine that developed over thousands of years by trial-and-error methods. Way back somewhere in prehistory, a medicine man or simply a venturesome sick person did some pricking with needles to see if pain could be alleviated or sickness cured.

The development of acupuncture into a full-fledged method of anesthesia for surgical operations did not take place during the long pre-Mao period of Chinese traditional medicine. It was a quite recent development, accomplished by medical researchers adapting traditional methods to the needs of modern, scientific medicine. Knowing the ability of acupuncture to control pain, they tried different needling points and techniques until they were able to so deaden pain that a person's abdominal cavity could be cut open and prolonged operations carried out with the patient feeling no pain, just a "heaviness" when the surgeon inserts his hand into the opening to examine various organs.

187

Needle anesthesia, which is the proper name for that technique, differs from acupuncture in that there is a strong emphasis on methods to increase the "energy" output of the needles by twirling, and even by electrical stimulation. Let me say here that no one—not even the obviously intelligent and well-trained Chinese surgeons and anesthetists whom we met in Shanghai—knows how to explain what makes this technique work. They have some pretty good ideas, but are still conducting research to try to pin down the scientific principles exactly.

The needle anesthetists apparently don't accept the traditional Chinese view that acupuncture needles interfere with flows of energy along the body's "meridians." Neither do they accept the view of some Western doctors that the effect is a form of hypnosis. They know through their experiments with animals that hypnosis does not play a part in the effect.

Ignorance of the exact fundamentals of the needling effect has not hindered the rapid development of the advanced techniques used in operations.

In the operation that I witnessed, the patient was anesthetized by six needles. Two were inserted in the abdomen, two in the back, and two in the left foot. Several of the needles were connected to a small electrical machine placed in back of the patient's head. A flashing light on the device indicated that pulsing energy was flowing into his body—I was told it was at the rate of 150 to 200 pulsations each minute at the very low rate of two milliamperes. I know that the electricity was going into the needle of the left foot, because I could see it jerking slightly in time with the pulses. (However, I don't recall that the foot was wiggling back and forth 150 times a minute. It seemed to me more like 70 or 80.)

Another difference between acupuncture and needle anesthesia is the length of time needed to get an effect. Acupuncture tends to be a relatively short-time thing, while needle anesthesia takes 30 minutes to become fully effective, I was told by Dr. Chin Hsiung-Yuan, the Chief Anesthetist of Hsinhua Hospital.

Timing is important in other ways in needle anesthesia. Not only must the patient be prepared according to schedule before the operation, but the work itself must be finished within the period that the anesthesia will be effective. Nervous energy, of a not completely explained form, is consumed to get the pain-deadening effect. During the most intensive portions of the operation, the electrical stimulation is greatest, so that the patient feels no pain. Chemical anesthesia is ready to be used if necessary. When the difficult part of the operation is completed, the electricity is turned low, or off altogether, as suturing is not as painful and can be completed without serious drains on the patient's nerve-energy stores.

Auricular Acupuncture

Most interesting to me was the massaging of the patient's ears that took place at the high points of the operation. The Chinese have discovered—apparently quite recently—that the ears are very sensitive and useful sites for anesthesia work and for acupuncture, and even for diagnosis of internal problems. They are perfecting a new science called "auricular acupuncture" (also under development in Germany and France) which may become very widely used in the West. I noticed that almost every drugstore in China today is selling plastic ears, numbered with acupuncture points, in the acupuncture needle section. A small instruction sheet—in Chinese, of course, —is supplied with the ear.

Then in Shanghai, at the large Friendship Store

catering to foreign visitors, I noticed that a small, electric device about the size of a pack of cigarettes was on sale next to the acupuncture dolls and needles. Curious, I asked the clerk about it and he explained that it is used to locate specific points on the ear which were linked to body organs. I questioned Dr. Chin about the auricular acupuncture technique and he said it does work, which is a convincing testimonial for me. He is an intelligent and capable physician.

Dr. Yo, the acupuncturist who treated my cold, said she also had one of the electrical auricular acupuncture devices and claimed it was useful, especially in diagnosing asthma cases. Since the small device allows the principles of acupuncture to be used without the need to prick the skin with needles, it could become quite popular here in the U.S., where a simpler, painless form of acupuncture would appeal to a wide audience.

Needle anesthesia is not effective for everyone. About 60 to 70 percent of people have good results. In China, the patient has the right to choose the method of anesthesia to be used, and obviously some people prefer to be put to sleep with chemical anesthesia. Apparently, though, the effectiveness of needle anesthesia doesn't depend on lifetime conditioning.

Some types of operations also preclude the use of needle anesthesia. Anesthesia (of any type) is usually less effective in "putting to sleep" the lower part of the body than the upper. Also, needle anesthesia doesn't work well for operations on children. Because the Hsinhua Hospital in Shanghai does a large amount of pediatric surgery, it ends up using needle anesthesia on only 30 percent of its surgical cases. The figure for other Chinese hospitals is probably higher.

Along about this time you might be asking yourself, "What's the whole point of needle anesthesia? Why not just let yourself be put out completely, in the American fashion?" The answer is that the needle way to deaden surgical pain has many important advantages. Chemical anesthesia can be quite a serious depressing force on the body's functions, and recovery from an operation is often as much recovery from the effects of chemical anesthesia as it is a healing process from the work of the knife. At the least, chemical anesthesia does take some "getting over" for a surgical patient.

Needle anesthesia, by contrast, allows the body to function in an almost completely normal way during surgery—a fact which has important advantages for the surgeon in some types of operations and for the patient in all cases. Mr. Chang, the surgical patient I was watching, maintained a normal pulse rate during the whole operation. It was eighty beats per minute the time I asked, at about the climax of the procedure. His blood pressure also stayed normal.

Experience has shown that people operated on under needle anesthesia recover more quickly than conventional surgical patients. We were told that recovery from an average type of operation takes 10 days when chemical anesthesia is used, and only 5 to 7 days after an operation done with needle anesthesia. Undoubtedly, there is a strong cost advantage in needle anesthesia. Needle treatment not only saves the expense of chemicals, but cuts down hospital occupancy rates and gets people back on the production line or to the farm commune faster.

After the major part of one operation I saw that used needle anesthesia, the patient was quite alert though slightly subdued. He did say that he "felt fairly well" and "expected to be back at work in half a month."

191

Will we ever be seeing needle anesthesia used for operations here? I think so, provided the heavy hand of unreasonable medical regulation doesn't get in the way of the experimentation and innovation needed.

Acupuncture without Needles

One way of using acupuncture points is now being done without needles.

In Japan, some physicians have achieved considerable success using simple thumb and hand pressure on the acupuncture points. The Japanese call it Shiatsu, which translated literally, means "finger pressure."

The Japanese Ministry of Welfare, which licenses practitioners, defines it as: "A treatment in which the thumbs and palms of the hands are used to apply pressure to certain points in order to correct irregularities of the living body, maintain or improve health, and contribute to the cure of certain illnesses."

Some of these illnesses that Shiatsu practitioners cure or improve include gastritis, fallen stomach, the common cold, toothache, headache, rheumatism, nose bleed, slipped disc and a variety of other problems.

As Shiatsu practitioners view it, pain induces muscular contractions in the affected area. A complicated chemical reaction continues to take place which only increases the pain. However, direct pressure over the spot causes the contractions to cease, eventually easing the pain too.

It sounds like a massage but it isn't. Shiatsu pressure is applied straight down with the balls of the thumb or, in the case of treatment to the eyes and abdomen, with the palm of the hand. Direct pressure of Shiatsu gives a much deeper and longer-lasting effect than a massage.

The Shiatsu manual points out that to "treat a specific illness, points nearest the ailing part demand attention, but sometimes pressure on distant areas brings greatest improvement. For instance, pressure is applied on the soles of the feet for kidney disease and to the left hand to strengthen the heart. Experience proclaims the efficacy of Shiatsu on apparently unrelated parts of the body, and factual medical cases substantiate it."

A dull and heavy head in the morning is attributed to a congestion of stale blood in the head area. Consequently, a Shiatsu treatment calls for stimulating a set of six pressure points in the head. The points run in a straight line from just above the nose to the center of the back of the head.

Using the bulb of the thumb, each of the points is pressed in turn and, it is said, that as you press these points on the crown of your head, you will notice that it begins to clear instantly.

The technique of the Shiatsu practitioner is to feel firmly around the locale of each of the points. When he hits the proper point, he recognizes it because he feels that it is more sensitive.

This treatment is then extended to the carotid artery which runs down the left and right sides of the neck. There are four pressure points that are stimulated for a second or two, first on the right and then on the left.

The whole treatment, which works for stiff neck or a hangover or that listless, mid-morning feeling of the "blah's," is designed to stimulate the flow of blood through the artery.

As in acupuncture, the hands—in particular the left—are presumed to be directly connected to the heart. The Nippon Shiatsu school claims that practicing Shiatsu, through its effect on the hands, strengthens the heart and other internal organs.

Does it work?

The writer of the Shiatsu manual claims that the technique can work apparent miracles because it takes advantage of the body's own wonderful natural powers. In other words, it is a technique entirely directed towards encouraging the body to heal itself.

There is an electronic theory of acupuncture. A French physician, Dr. Georges Cantoni, has found that people have a different electrical potential in their heads than they do in their fingertips. The difference can be thirty to forty millivolts. When health is poor, this electric difference can be mixed up. The Chinese talk about the circulation of energy in the body as being a vital part of acupuncture theory.

That leads us to the possibility that there are other ways than acupuncture to put the body's electronic potential back in shape. For example, many people have reported that they feel better when walking barefoot on bare earth than they do while on concrete, or in steel-framed buildings.

Up to now, those claims have been dismissed as irrational. But if acupuncture is shown to achieve its remarkable effects through electronic means, perhaps walking barefoot on the earth will someday be investigated too. That could lead to a new trend toward natural living, with a scientific basis in fact.

Weird Ideas Worth Exploring

Here are some other seemingly weird ideas that are worth exploring, in the light of the acupuncture revelation:

People can talk to their organs. An aged friend

told me a few years back that he communicated with his liver and gall bladder every night before going to sleep. He did it by sending calming thoughts to those parts of his body. Exactly what he said to his organs he didn't reveal, but he was the picture of health.

I thought he was kidding me. Then not long afterward I saw in a scientific journal that young volunteers were being taught to lower their blood pressure by mental training. Even experimental animals have been taught the technique, called visceral learning.

Eventually, people may be trained to control a variety of chronic diseases without the use of expensive and possibly harmful drugs. All they'll have to do is learn to think themselves healthy. It's weird, but it does work.

Plants have prejudices, just like people. Many gardeners are now using companion planting methods. They put pumpkins next to corn because folklore tells them that those two plants are happier together. Other vegetables also ward off insects and disease better when planted together.

Some plant friendships have been proven by research. It is known that plants send out airborne hormones—called pheromones—which can influence the behavior of insects. That may explain plant friendships and antagonisms. The pheromones from one kind of plant may drive away enemies of other plants.

Commercial farmers still scorn companion planting, just as Western doctors avoided acupuncture for many years. They use large amounts of pesticides to control insects and diseases that might be limited through companion planting. Even fertilizer use could possibly be cut by putting friendly plants together.

Some scientists are trying to carry plant "friendships" to extremes. They are attempting to merge the germ cells of wheat and a legume to produce a grain plant that will be able to capture nitrogen from the air. That could cut the need for nitrogen fertilizer.

Natural foods have a spark of life that is removed by processing. That idea has been around as long as people have been making white flour and polished rice. Some people just feel better and healthier when they are eating whole foods, and claim that there is a real basis for their euphoria.

German food enthusiasts even claim that whole wheat flour loses its spark of life within twenty-four hours of milling. They grind grain every day in handmills, and always use it fresh.

There is some evidence to support claims of an X-factor in whole foods. Experimental animals fed ground whole wheat were found able to withstand otherwise fatal doses of typhoid germs. That was reported by Dr. Howard A. Schneider in the November 3, 1967 issue of *Science.* He said the factor responsible is in the bran-germ part of the wheat, and called it pacifarin.

Until recently, strange ideas have been automatically rejected by most scientists. Now the climate is changing. There's a growing feeling that conventional science has built-in blind spots that leave some useful techniques undiscovered.

Most unorthodox techniques are hard to prove valuable. Long-term and highly complex experiments would have to be conducted to explain how and why effects are achieved. And since there is usually no product to be sold, money to support that research is hard to find.

Electrical energy may play a major role in our future health program. Try to imagine a time in the not too distant future when many of the everyday ills that beset us—from sprained ankles and insomnia to fractured ribs and damaged hearts—will be routinely healed by small surges of electrical energy. That certainly sounds far out now, but preliminary tests have excited the medical community about the potential of electricity as a healing agent.

"We are on the threshold of a new era in medicine in which bioelectronics offers the clinician control over basic life processes which even a decade ago could not have been anticipated," predicts Dr. Robert O. Becker of Veterans Administration Hospital in Syracuse, New York. After 15 years of investigation, Dr. Becker is convinced that life at the cellular level is regulated by naturally-occurring electronic impulses, so weak they've gone unmeasured until quite recently. He says he's seen the response to his work change "from complete rejection just over a decade ago through amused disbelief to—at present—enthusiastic acceptance."

Amputated forelimbs of 21-day-old white rats have been partially regrown when low levels of direct current were applied by Dr. Becker. Although the limbs were not completely restored (as a salamander is able to do), bone cartilage, bone marrow, nerve, muscle and blood vessels all were regenerated to a certain extent.

There are already a number of ways that electromagnetic energy is being used to help human beings:

Bone fractures. Orthopedic surgeons at the University of Pennsylvania have successfully healed stubborn fractures with electricity.

Anesthesia. In clinical trials, low-level electrical energy has induced general anesthesia (electronarcosis) and regional anesthesia when used in conjunction with acupuncture.

Insomnia. Researchers are trying to learn more about possible applications of alternating current to produce sleep. Electrosleep therapy is being used at the University of California at San Diego to treat patients with chronic anxiety.

Local healing. Electricity speeds healing of skin ulcers and burns. British surgeon D. H. Wilson has reported significant reduction in pain and disability among sprained-ankle patients treated with pulsed electrical energy.

Eventually, such therapy may even be prescribed for heart attack victims. "If we could gain access to these (electrical) control systems in an effective fashion," Dr. Becker suggested in *Technology Review* (December, 1972) "we would be able to bring about the repair of damaged heart muscle by growing new heart muscle instead of scar."

The notion that all living things are somehow affected by an invisible flux of minute electrical energy should come as no surprise. We're all familiar with the unseen force that causes compass needles to spin, but what about these verified (but unexplained) phenomena:

Disturbances in the earth's magnetic field caused by magnetic storms and solar eruptions are statistically linked to human behavior disturbances.

Birds and other migrating animals somehow use the planet's electromagnetic field to navigate.

Past reversals of the earth's field have been associated with the extinction of certain species of wildlife.

Are we heading into a new age, where results count for more than neat logic? That's quite possible, and it could open the doors to other changes in the way people live, eat, and are treated for illness.

Index